Medical Billing Denials Decoded

The Insider's Playbook for Fixing Claims, Cutting Rejections, and Getting Paid Faster

Ryan Mitchell, MD

Table of Content

CHAPTER 1 11
The Revenue Cycle in One Page
CHAPTER 2 20
Code Systems Without the Overwhelm
CHAPTER 3 32
Reading an Explanation of Benefits Like a Pro
CHAPTER 4 52
Eligibility and Coverage Denials
CHAPTER 5 63
Duplicate Claim Denials
CHAPTER 6 75
Prior Authorization Denials
CHAPTER 7 87
Medical Necessity Denials
CHAPTER 8 100
Timely Filing Denials
CHAPTER 9 112
Modifier and Coding Denials
CHAPTER 10 125
Demographic and Data Entry Denials
CHAPTER 11 137
The 90-Day Appeal Master Plan
CHAPTER 12 150
Denial Rate Benchmarks and KPIs That Matter
CHAPTER 13 160
Modifiers Quick-Reference and Cheat Sheets
CHAPTER 14 178
Remote Work and Career Path in Medical Billing

INTRODUCTION

Why Claims Get Denied (and Why No One Tells You)

The industry's dirty secret — most denials are preventable

You submitted the claim correctly. The patient was seen, the service was documented, the code matched the diagnosis, and the charge went out on time. Two weeks later: denied.

No explanation you can act on. A reason code that tells you the claim was denied but not why it was really denied or what to do about it. A phone number that puts you on hold for 45 minutes before disconnecting. And a growing stack of the same problem waiting on your desk.

If that sounds familiar, you already know the thing this book is about. What you may not know is how predictable it all is — and how fixable.

The Number Nobody Mentions

The U.S. healthcare system processes approximately 3 billion medical claims per year. Of those, an estimated 15 to 20 percent are initially denied by payers. That is somewhere between 450 million and 600 million rejected claims every year.

$262B

in claims denied annually in the U.S. healthcare system

Source: American Medical Association, 2023 AMA Prior Authorization Survey and claims data

What makes that number extraordinary is what the research consistently shows underneath it: the majority of those denials are preventable. Studies by the Medical Group Management Association (MGMA) and the American Academy of Family Physicians (AAFP) have found that between 65 and 75 percent of denied claims could have been avoided with different front-end processes, correct coding the first time, or proper documentation at the point of care.

> *Between 65 and 75 percent of denied claims could have been avoided. Not appealed and won later — avoided entirely.*

This book is not about accepting that number. It is about dismantling it.

Why Nobody Tells You

Here is the part that takes most people in this industry a few years to figure out: the system does not particularly want you to understand why claims get denied.

Payers profit from denials. Not because they are malicious, but because their processes are designed to move fast, and the path of least resistance is to deny first and wait to see if the provider bothers to appeal. Approximately 60 percent of denied claims are never appealed at all. Of the ones that are appealed, around 65 percent are eventually overturned in the provider's favor. Read those two numbers together and you will understand the business logic on the payer side.

Medical schools do not teach billing. Nursing programs do not teach billing. Even many coding certification programs teach you how to assign a code but spend surprisingly little time on what happens when that coded claim gets rejected and you have to fight for the money. The assumption is that you will learn it on the job.

And you do learn it on the job. The problem is that learning it on the job takes years, costs your practice significant revenue during those years, and relies almost entirely on whoever happens to be sitting next to you and willing to share what they know.

This book is an attempt to compress that learning curve significantly.

The Six Root Causes of Claim Denials

In a moment we will get into the specific denial types and how to fix each one. But before that, it is worth understanding that virtually every denial in medical billing traces back to one of six root causes. Knowing the root cause before you look at a denial code tells you which part of your process failed — and which part you need to fix to stop it from happening again.

#	Root Cause	What It Means in Practice
1	**Patient eligibility**	The patient's coverage was not active, not applicable to the service, or was verified incorrectly at check-in. The claim was dead before it left the office.
2	**Missing or incorrect authorization**	The service required prior authorization that was not obtained, or was obtained for the wrong service, wrong date, or wrong facility.

3	**Coding errors**	The procedure code, diagnosis code, or modifier was incorrect, missing, or failed to meet the payer's coverage criteria for that combination.
4	**Documentation gaps**	The clinical documentation in the record does not support the level of service billed or the medical necessity of the procedure.
5	**Administrative / data errors**	Name spelled wrong, date of birth entered incorrectly, NPI missing, claim submitted to the wrong payer, or a dozen other entry-level mistakes that should not exist but do.
6	**Timely filing**	The claim was submitted outside the payer's allowed window. This denial is almost always 100 percent preventable and always 100 percent the biller's responsibility.

Every chapter in Part 2 of this book addresses one or more of these root causes. By the time you finish Part 2, you will be able to look at any denial and immediately identify not just the fix but the underlying process failure that allowed it to happen.

What This Book Is and Is Not

What it is

- A practical reference for medical billers, billing managers, front desk staff, and practice managers who deal with denied claims in their daily work.
- A focused guide to the most common denial types — not an attempt to cover every possible scenario in the entire history of claims processing.
- A system for prevention, not just repair. Each denial chapter gives you the fix for today and the workflow change that stops the same denial from coming back next month.
- A career resource for people who are new to medical billing and want to understand how the industry actually works before they are sitting in front of a denial queue on their first week.

What it is not

- A coding manual. This book does not teach you to assign ICD-10 or CPT codes from scratch. Chapter 2 covers the code systems at the level of understanding you need to troubleshoot denials, but if you need a comprehensive coding reference, you will want a dedicated resource for that.
- A payer-specific guide. Every major payer — UnitedHealthcare, Aetna, BCBS, Cigna, Humana, Medicare, Medicaid — has its own policies and quirks. This book covers the denial types that apply across payers, with notes on where payer-specific rules are particularly important.
- A substitute for your payer contracts. The rules that govern what you can and cannot bill are ultimately in your contracts. This book gives you the tools to work those contracts effectively.

How to Use This Book

The chapters in this book are designed so that you can read it straight through or jump to the specific denial type you are dealing with right now.

> **IF YOU ARE NEW TO MEDICAL BILLING:** Read Part 1 (Chapters 1-3) before anything else. These three chapters give you the foundation that makes everything in Part 2 make sense. They are written to be read in about two hours and will save you weeks of confusion on the job.

> **IF YOU ARE AN EXPERIENCED BILLER:** Go directly to the denial chapter in Part 2 that matches the problem you are trying to solve right now. Each chapter is self-contained. Use the quick-reference index at the back of the book to find a specific denial code fast.

IF YOU ARE A BILLING MANAGER OR PRACTICE OWNER: Part 3 is where you want to focus after getting oriented in Part 1. The KPI chapter, the denial dashboard template, and the workflow audit tools in Part 3 are designed for the person responsible for the system, not just the individual claims.

BEFORE WE START: A REALISTIC EXPECTATION

This book will not eliminate every denial in your practice. Some denials will always happen — payer systems change, contracts get renegotiated, and physicians occasionally document things in ways that create billing challenges no system can fully prevent.

What this book will do: give you a clear, actionable response to the denials you see most often, and a set of front-end processes that measurably reduces how often those denials appear in the first place. Practices that implement the prevention workflows in this book consistently achieve first-pass claim rates of 95 percent or higher. The national average is around 85 percent. That gap represents real money.

The Vocabulary You Will Need

A few terms appear throughout this book that are worth defining upfront. These are not definitions for their own sake — they are the specific way these terms are used in this book, which sometimes differs slightly from how you might see them used in other contexts.

Term	How It Is Used in This Book
Denial	A claim that has been adjudicated and rejected by the payer. Distinct from a rejection (which is a claim returned before adjudication for technical errors) and a pending claim (which is still being processed).
Rejection	A claim returned before adjudication, usually for technical errors like a missing NPI or a name mismatch. Rejections are fixed and resubmitted; denials are appealed.

Adjustment reason code	The code on the explanation of benefits (EOB) or remittance advice (ERA) that identifies the reason for the denial or payment reduction. CO, PR, and OA are the three main prefixes.
Remark code	A secondary code on the EOB that adds detail to the adjustment reason code. MA, N, and M series codes. Often more actionable than the reason code alone.
First-pass rate	The percentage of claims that are paid on the first submission without requiring any follow-up, correction, or appeal. The primary KPI for billing efficiency.
Clean claim	A claim submitted without errors that is adjudicated within the payer's standard processing time. A clean claim is not necessarily a paid claim — it can be cleanly denied.
Appeal	A formal request to reconsider a denied claim. Appeals have defined timeframes, documentation requirements, and escalation levels depending on the payer and the denial type.

> *The goal is not to win every denial fight. It is to build a system where most of the fights never start.*

Let's get started.

CHAPTER 1
The Revenue Cycle in One Page

The entire billing workflow without the textbook treatment

Most billing textbooks spend thirty to fifty pages explaining the revenue cycle. By page twenty you are memorizing org charts. By page forty you have forgotten what you were reading.

This chapter does it differently. The revenue cycle is eight steps. Each step has an owner, a job, and a specific place where denials are born. You can understand the whole thing in the time it takes to drink a cup of coffee. What you do with that understanding is what the rest of this book is about.

The Eight Steps — and Where Denials Are Born

Every claim that your practice submits has traveled through a sequence of steps before it arrives at the payer. Each step is a handoff. Each handoff is a point where information can be incomplete, incorrect, or missing. Denials are almost always the downstream consequence of something that went wrong at one of these eight steps.

1

Patient Scheduling and Registration

Who: Front desk / patient access team

The patient's demographics, insurance information, and referring provider details are collected. This is the first point of contact between the patient and the billing system.

⚠ **Denial risk:** *Name misspellings, wrong date of birth, incorrect subscriber ID, and wrong insurance carrier account for 15-20% of all administrative denials. The data entered here flows into every step that follows.*

2

Insurance Eligibility Verification

Who: Front desk / billing team

The patient's insurance is confirmed as active and applicable to the scheduled service before the appointment occurs. This includes confirming the plan type, deductible status, copay amounts, and any benefit limits.

⚠ **Denial risk:** *Failure to verify, or verifying but not checking the specific service, is the root cause of CO-31 (patient not eligible) and CO-4 (service not covered) denials. Eligibility verified yesterday does not mean eligible today.*

3

Prior Authorization (when required)

Who: Billing team / clinical staff

For services that require advance payer approval, the authorization is obtained before the appointment. This involves submitting clinical criteria to the payer and receiving a reference number that is attached to the claim.

⚠ **Denial risk:** *No authorization, wrong authorization for the actual service rendered, or expired authorization accounts for a significant portion of the most expensive denials. See Chapter 6 for the full prior auth framework.*

4

Patient Encounter and Documentation

Who: Physician / clinical staff

The patient is seen. The physician documents the visit, procedures performed, and diagnoses in the medical record. The documentation here is the legal and clinical foundation of everything that follows in billing.

⚠ **Denial risk:** *Insufficient documentation to support the level of service billed, or a diagnosis that does not clearly link to the procedure performed, is the root cause of medical necessity denials (CO-50, CO-57). No biller can fix documentation that the physician did not write.*

5

Charge Capture and Coding

Who: Coder / billing team

The clinical documentation is translated into billable codes: ICD-10 diagnosis codes, CPT procedure codes, and modifiers where applicable. Charges are entered into the practice management system.

⚠ **Denial risk:** *Wrong code, missing modifier, incorrect code pairing, or a code that has been updated since the coder last checked is the root cause of CO-4, CO-11, CO-22, and most bundling denials. This is where most experienced billers focus their quality control.*

6

Claim Submission

Who: Billing team / clearinghouse

The coded claim is transmitted electronically to the payer, usually through a clearinghouse that validates the claim format before forwarding it. The clearinghouse performs technical edits (format, required fields) but does not check clinical accuracy.

⚠ **Denial risk:** *Claims rejected at this stage are technical rejections, not clinical denials — they come back before adjudication. Common: missing NPI, incorrect taxonomy code, claim format errors. Fix and resubmit, usually within 24-48 hours.*

7

Payer Adjudication

Who: Payer (insurance company)

The payer reviews the claim against the patient's plan benefits, the provider's contract, clinical coverage policies, and any flags from automated editing systems. The claim is approved, partially approved, or denied.

⚠ **Denial risk:** *This is where most formal denials are generated. The denial reason code on the EOB identifies the official reason, but the real cause almost always traces back to one of the earlier steps. The payer is surfacing a problem that already existed.*

8

Payment Posting, Follow-Up, and Appeals

Who: Billing team

Payments are posted to patient accounts. Denials are reviewed and routed to the correct team member for appeal or write-off. The aging report is monitored for claims that have not been paid within the expected timeframe.

> ⚠ **Denial risk:** *This is where revenue is recovered or lost. Practices that do not have a systematic follow-up process for denied claims leave significant money on the table. Most payers allow 30 to 180 days from the denial date to submit an appeal.*

Where Denials Actually Enter the Cycle

The claim is denied at Step 7. But the denial was caused at Step 1, 2, 3, 4, or 5. This is the most important distinction in all of medical billing, and most denial management processes get it backwards — they spend all their energy on Step 8 (appealing the denial) while the same error continues to occur at Step 1 through 5 every day.

Denial Shows Up	But Was Caused At	What That Means for Prevention
Step 7 (Adjudication)	**Step 1-2 (Registration/Eligibility)**	Fix the front-end process: verify eligibility more thoroughly, update registration workflows, catch insurance changes before the claim goes out.
Step 7 (Adjudication)	**Step 3 (Prior Auth)**	Fix the authorization tracking system: know which services require auth, build a tracking log, verify auth before every appointment for affected services.
Step 7 (Adjudication)	**Step 4 (Documentation)**	This requires provider engagement: feedback loops, documentation templates, or clinical documentation improvement (CDI) programs. The biller cannot fix this alone.

Step 7 (Adjudication)	**Step 5 (Coding)**	Fix the coding process: coder training, annual CPT updates, modifier decision trees, internal audits. The most controllable denial category.
Step 7 (Adjudication)	**Step 6 (Submission)**	Fix the clearinghouse edit setup and claim scrubbing rules. Most of these are technical and systematic, not clinical.

> *Appealing a denial fixes this claim. Finding where in the cycle the error occurred fixes the next hundred claims.*

The Players — Who Does What

One of the most common sources of confusion for people new to medical billing is understanding which person or system is responsible for which part of the process. The same title means different things in different practice settings, and the same task can belong to different people depending on whether you are in a solo practice, a physician group, or a hospital system.

The following descriptions are based on the most common division of responsibilities in a small to mid-size physician practice. Use this as a reference for understanding who to work with when a specific denial needs to be addressed.

Player	Primary Role in Revenue Cycle	Where They Affect Denials
Front desk / patient access	Registration, eligibility verification, copay collection, scheduling	Steps 1 and 2. Errors here produce administrative denials (wrong name, wrong insurance, eligibility not verified). The first and most preventable source of denials.
Medical coder	Translates clinical documentation into ICD-10, CPT, and HCPCS codes	Step 5. Coding errors produce CO-4, CO-11, CO-22, and bundling denials. The most technically complex source of denials.
Medical biller	Submits claims, posts payments, follows up on denials, manages aging	Steps 6 and 8. The biller is the last line of defense before submission and the first responder when denials arrive.
Clinical staff / physician	Documents the encounter in the medical record	Step 4. Documentation gaps produce medical necessity denials. Billers cannot create documentation — they can only work with what exists.
Billing manager / practice manager	Oversees the entire revenue cycle, sets KPIs, handles payer relations	All steps. Responsible for the system that prevents denials, not individual claim fixes.
Clearinghouse	Electronic transmission and technical validation of claims	Step 6. Acts as a filter between the practice and the payer. Returns claims with format errors before adjudication.

Payer (insurance)	Adjudicates claims against plan benefits and coverage policies	Step 7. Issues the denial with a reason code. The payer is the endpoint, not the origin, of most denial problems.

What Billers Actually Control — and What They Don't

This is a distinction worth making explicit because a significant amount of billing frustration comes from taking responsibility for problems that originated in someone else's part of the process.

The Biller Controls	The Biller Does NOT Control
Claim accuracy before submission	What the physician documented in the chart
Modifier application	Whether the diagnosis clinically supports the procedure
Timely filing — completely within the biller's lane	Whether the payer's coverage policies are reasonable
Eligibility verification (if it's in their workflow)	What the payer decides during adjudication
Following up on unpaid and denied claims	The front desk's accuracy in capturing patient demographics
Writing and submitting appeals	Whether the physician obtained prior authorization
Monitoring the aging report	Payer contract terms (negotiated by the practice owner or administrator)
Identifying patterns in denials	Clinical staff's documentation completeness

WHY THIS MATTERS: When a biller takes ownership of denials that originated in a part of the process they cannot control — physician documentation, front desk registration errors, prior auth failures — the result is exhaustion without resolution. The correct response to those denials is to identify the root cause, communicate it to the person who controls that step, and help build a fix. Not to absorb the problem personally.

The Three Points Where Most Denials Originate

You now have the full eight-step picture. In practice, the data consistently points to three of those eight steps as the origin of the vast majority of denials:

POINT 1 — ELIGIBILITY AND REGISTRATION (Steps 1-2)

Approximately 23-27% of all denials originate here. Patient demographics entered incorrectly, insurance not verified before the visit, coverage terminated between verification and service date, wrong insurance plan on file. All of these are preventable with the right front-end workflow.

POINT 2 — PRIOR AUTHORIZATION (Step 3)

Approximately 11-15% of denials by count, but a disproportionately high percentage by dollar value because the services requiring prior auth tend to be higher-cost procedures, imaging, and specialist referrals. These denials are almost always completely preventable.

POINT 3 — CODING AND CHARGE CAPTURE (Step 5)

Approximately 25-30% of denials originate from coding errors. This is the highest-value target for a biller because it is the step most directly within billing's control and the step most responsive to training, auditing, and systematic correction.

The Takeaway From This Chapter

The revenue cycle is not complicated once you see it as a flow rather than a list of tasks. Eight steps, eight handoffs, eight places where something can go wrong. The denial arrives at Step 7 but the problem was born somewhere in Steps 1 through 5.

When you get a denial, your first question is not: how do I appeal this? Your first question is: at which step did the information fail? That question tells you which process to fix, which person to talk to, and whether this denial is likely to keep happening until something upstream changes.

The chapters that follow will give you the specific answer for each denial type you are most likely to encounter. Keep the eight steps in mind as you read them. Every fix in this book is ultimately a fix to one of those eight steps.

> *The denial arrives at Step 7. But Step 7 has never been the problem.*

CHAPTER 2
Code Systems Without the Overwhelm

ICD-10, CPT, HCPCS, and modifiers — just what you need

Every denied claim has a code at the center of it. The code was missing, or wrong, or used in a combination the payer won't accept, or outdated by a year because nobody checked the annual updates. You don't need to know every code in existence to fix that. You need to understand how the code systems work — well enough to spot the problem and know where to look.

This chapter covers ICD-10, CPT, and HCPCS at the level of understanding that matters for denial management. Not as a coding course. Not as an exam prep guide. As the foundation you need to understand why a claim was denied and what it will take to fix it.

ICD-10: The Diagnosis Code

ICD-10 stands for International Classification of Diseases, 10th Revision. In the United States, we use ICD-10-CM (Clinical Modification), which is the version adapted for outpatient and physician billing. The ICD-10 code tells the payer why the patient was seen — the medical reason that justifies the service.

How an ICD-10 Code Is Built

Every ICD-10-CM code follows a predictable structure. Once you understand the structure, you can read any code you have never seen before and know which body system and category it belongs to.

M54.51

M — Chapter/body system — M = Musculoskeletal system and connective tissue
54 — Category — 54 = Dorsalgia (back pain)
51 — Subcategory/specificity — 51 = Vertebrogenic low back pain

ICD-10-CM codes are 3 to 7 characters long. The first character is always a letter. Characters 2 and 3 are numbers. Characters 4 through 7 (if present) provide additional specificity: laterality (right vs left), episode of care (initial vs subsequent vs sequela), or further clinical detail.

The ICD-10 Rules That Cause Denials

- Code to the highest level of specificity: if a 7-character code exists for the condition, submitting a 5-character version will trigger a CO-4 denial (service inconsistent with the procedure). Payers require the most specific code available.
- Use current codes: ICD-10-CM is updated annually on October 1. A code that was valid last year may be deleted, split, or revised this year. Using a deleted code triggers a technical rejection or a CO-4 denial. Build an annual code update review into your October workflow.
- The diagnosis must support the procedure: the ICD-10 code submitted with a CPT code must logically and clinically justify that service. A diagnosis of J00 (common cold) submitted with CPT 71046 (chest X-ray, 2 views) will trigger a medical necessity denial (CO-50) from most payers. The link between why the patient was seen and what was done is not optional.
- Unspecified codes: codes ending in -9 or labeled 'unspecified' are acceptable when the clinical information genuinely does not support a more specific code. Using them when a more specific code exists — or as a shortcut — increases denial and audit risk.

> **THE MOST COMMON ICD-10 DENIAL TRIGGER:** Submitting a code that exists but does not support the procedure billed. The code is real, it is valid, it is not deleted — it just does not give the payer a reason to pay for what was done. This is a linking problem, not a code lookup problem. The solution is in the documentation and in the coder's understanding of the clinical connection.

CPT: The Procedure Code

CPT stands for Current Procedural Terminology. It is published and maintained by the American Medical Association (AMA) and updated annually. CPT codes describe what was done to the patient — the service, procedure, or test that was performed.

Every CPT code is a 5-digit number. The codes are organized into six sections:

Code Range	Section	What It Covers
99202-99499	**Evaluation and Management (E/M)**	Office visits, hospital visits, consultations, preventive medicine. The most frequently billed section in outpatient medicine.
00100-01999	**Anesthesia**	Anesthesia services for surgical procedures. Uses a different payment calculation (base units + time units).
10004-69990	**Surgery**	Surgical procedures across all body systems. Includes the global surgical package concept that causes many modifier denials.

70010-79999	**Radiology**	Diagnostic imaging and radiation therapy. Includes professional and technical component billing (modifiers 26 and TC).
80047-89398	**Pathology and Laboratory**	Lab tests, pathology interpretations, genetic testing. High volume in primary care and specialist settings.
90281-99607	**Medicine**	Vaccines, injections, psychiatry, physical therapy, dialysis, and miscellaneous services that do not fit other sections.

E/M Codes: The Most Billed and Most Audited

Evaluation and Management codes are the codes attached to office visits and most outpatient encounters. If your practice does any primary care, internal medicine, or outpatient specialty care, you will encounter E/M codes daily. They are also the codes most frequently targeted in payer audits.

E/M codes are selected based on two factors: medical decision making (MDM) or total time spent with the patient on the date of service. The 2021 E/M revisions simplified the selection criteria significantly, but MDM documentation is still where most E/M denials originate — specifically, documentation that does not support the complexity level billed.

Code	Level	Time (typical)	MDM Complexity Required
99202	New patient — 2	15-29 min	Straightforward: minor or self-limited problem, minimal data review, minimal risk
99203	New patient — 3	30-44 min	Low complexity: low risk, limited data, 2+ self-limited problems or 1 stable chronic condition

99204	New patient — 4	45-59 min	Moderate complexity: multiple chronic conditions or new problem with additional workup, prescription drug management
99205	New patient — 5	60-74 min	High complexity: severe exacerbation, drug therapy requiring intensive monitoring, or decision regarding hospitalization
99213	Est. patient — 3	20-29 min	Low complexity: same criteria as new patient low
99214	Est. patient — 4	30-39 min	Moderate complexity: same criteria as new patient moderate
99215	Est. patient — 5	40-54 min	High complexity: same criteria as new patient high

The Global Surgical Package

When a surgical CPT code is billed, it includes a bundle of pre-operative, intra-operative, and post-operative services. This is the global surgical package. Understanding it prevents modifier denials.

- 0-day global period: minor procedures where the day of surgery and any related E/M on the same day are included. Billing a separate office visit on the day of a minor procedure requires modifier 25 on the E/M.
- 10-day global period: the day of surgery plus 10 days of routine follow-up care. Billing a separate E/M within this window requires modifier 24 (unrelated condition) or 79 (unrelated procedure).
- 90-day global period: the day before surgery, the day of surgery, and 90 days of routine post-operative care. This applies to most major surgical procedures. Billing a separate E/M for a related condition within this 90-day window without a modifier will result in a bundling denial.

HCPCS Level II: When CPT Isn't Enough

HCPCS (pronounced 'hick-picks') stands for Healthcare Common Procedure Coding System. Level I of HCPCS is CPT. Level II is a separate set of codes maintained by the Centers for Medicare and Medicaid Services (CMS) for items and services that CPT does not cover.

HCPCS Level II codes are one letter followed by four numbers (for example, J0696 for ceftriaxone injection, L1832 for a knee orthosis, or A6216 for a gauze dressing). They are used primarily for:

- Injectable drugs and biologics (J-codes)
- Durable medical equipment, prosthetics, orthotics, and supplies (DMEPOS)
- Ambulance and transportation services
- Dental procedures (D-codes)
- Temporary codes assigned by CMS for emerging services not yet in CPT

> **WHEN DO YOU NEED HCPCS LEVEL II?** If you are billing for drugs administered in the office (including chemotherapy, infusions, and injections), durable medical equipment, or supply items, HCPCS Level II codes are required rather than optional. Submitting a CPT code for a service that requires a HCPCS code — or submitting no code at all — will result in a denial or non-payment. Check payer policies, as some commercial payers use different coding conventions from Medicare for the same service.

The Ten Modifiers That Cause 80% of Modifier Denials

Modifiers are two-character codes (numeric or alphanumeric) appended to a CPT or HCPCS code to tell the payer that a service was altered in some way from its standard description — without changing the fundamental definition of the code itself. When used correctly, modifiers prevent denials. When missing or misapplied, they cause them.

The following ten modifiers account for the vast majority of modifier-related denials in outpatient physician billing. Each is presented with its intended use, a real-world example, and the most common mistake that produces a denial.

-25

Significant, Separately Identifiable E/M Service

Use when: A significant and separately identifiable E/M service was provided on the same day as a procedure or other service by the same physician.

Example: *Patient comes in for a wart removal (17110). During the same visit, the physician evaluates and documents a new diagnosis of hypertension. Bill 17110 and 99213-25.*

⚠ **Common trap:** Using -25 on every E/M regardless of whether a truly separate service was documented. Payers increasingly audit -25 usage. The documentation must show that the E/M was distinct from the pre-procedure assessment.

-51

Multiple Procedures

Use when: Multiple procedures, other than E/M services, were performed at the same session by the same provider.

Example: *A physician performs two separate surgical procedures in the same operative session. The primary procedure is billed without -51. The secondary procedure is billed with -51 to indicate a reduced fee applies.*

⚠ **Common trap:** Applying -51 to codes that are in the Medicare Multiple Procedure Payment Reduction (MPPR) category and have their own built-in reduction. Some payers exempt -51 entirely — know your payer's rules before appending it.

-59

Distinct Procedural Service

Use when: A procedure or service was distinct or independent from other services performed on the same day. Used to indicate that a service is not a component of another service.

Example: *A physician performs a service that would normally be bundled with another service billed on the same day, but it was performed at a different site, different session, or for a different injury.*

⚠ **Common trap:** Overusing -59 to unbundle codes that are legitimately bundled. CMS and most payers scrutinize -59 heavily. If a more specific modifier (XE, XS, XP, XU) applies, use it instead of -59.

-24

Unrelated E/M During Postoperative Period

Use when: An E/M service was provided during the postoperative period for a reason unrelated to the original procedure.

Example: *A patient who had knee surgery 30 days ago comes in reporting new chest pain. The physician evaluates the chest pain. Bill the E/M with -24 to indicate it is unrelated to the surgical global period.*

⚠ **Common trap:** Using -24 for follow-up care that IS related to the original surgery. The documentation must clearly show that the visit was for a separate, unrelated problem. Payers will request records.

-76

Repeat Procedure by Same Physician

Use when: A procedure or service was repeated by the same physician or other qualified health care professional subsequent to the original procedure or service.

Example: *A chest X-ray is taken in the morning and repeated in the afternoon of the same day to assess a change in condition. Both are billed — the second with -76.*

⚠ **Common trap:** Confusing -76 (same physician repeats) with -77 (different physician repeats). Using the wrong modifier produces a bundling denial even though the repeat procedure is clinically legitimate.

-77

Repeat Procedure by Another Physician

Use when: A procedure or service was repeated by a different physician than the one who originally performed it.

Example: *One radiologist reads the morning chest X-ray. A different radiologist reads the afternoon repeat. The second reading is billed with -77 to indicate a different provider performed it.*

⚠ **Common trap:** Same as -76: using -76 when the procedure was repeated by a different physician, or vice versa. The physician identity determines which modifier applies.

-79

Unrelated Procedure During Postoperative Period

Use when: A procedure performed during the postoperative period was unrelated to the original procedure.

Example: *A patient in a 90-day global period for a knee replacement fractures their wrist and requires surgical repair. The wrist surgery is billed with -79 to indicate it is unrelated to the knee procedure.*

⚠ **Common trap:** Failing to append -79 when performing a legitimately unrelated procedure in a global period. Without this modifier, the second procedure will be denied as included in the global surgical package.

-26

Professional Component

Use when: Only the professional component of a service was provided (the physician interpretation), not the technical component.

Example: *A radiologist interprets an X-ray taken at a hospital facility. The radiologist bills the CPT code with -26 to claim only the reading fee, not the facility fee for the equipment and staff.*

⚠ **Common trap:** Billing the full CPT code without -26 when only the professional component was provided. This causes a duplicate billing denial or overpayment recovery because the facility billed the TC component separately.

-TC

Technical Component

Use when: Only the technical component of a service was provided (the facility, equipment, and staff), not the professional component.

Example: *A hospital outpatient department performs an X-ray but contracts with an independent radiology group for interpretations. The hospital bills CPT with -TC for the equipment and staff portion.*

⚠ **Common trap:** Billing TC without confirming the professional component is being billed separately by another provider. If both components are billed by the same provider, neither modifier is used — the full code is billed.

-GT

Via Interactive Audio and Video

Use when: Services were rendered via real-time interactive audio and video telecommunications technology (telehealth).

Example: *A physician conducts a telehealth visit with an established patient. The E/M code is billed with -GT to indicate the service was delivered via video.*

⚠ **Common trap:** Confirming payer acceptance of -GT vs the newer GQ (store-and-forward) modifier, and verifying telehealth coverage for the specific service under the patient's plan. Coverage varies significantly by payer and state.

The Annual Update: Why October Matters

CPT codes are updated every January 1. ICD-10-CM codes are updated every October 1. Missing an annual update is one of the most preventable and most common sources of coding denials.

ANNUAL CODE UPDATE CHECKLIST

January 1 — CPT updates:

- Review the AMA's summary of new, deleted, and revised codes
- Update your practice management system's code tables before the first claim of the new year
- Check that any fee schedule changes affecting your most-used codes have been updated

October 1 — ICD-10-CM updates:

- Review the CMS ICD-10-CM update summary (available free at cms.gov)

- Flag any deleted codes that your practice uses frequently and identify their replacements
- Update your EHR's diagnosis code picklists — particularly for your top 20 most-used diagnoses
- Notify clinical staff of any documentation changes required to support new specificity requirements

The Code-Denial Connection

Now that you understand how each system works, here is the map of which denial codes you will encounter when each system fails:

Code System	Common Denial Code	Plain-English Meaning
ICD-10 (wrong or missing)	**CO-4**	The procedure code is inconsistent with the diagnosis code submitted. The most common version: the diagnosis does not clinically justify the service.
ICD-10 (deleted code)	**CO-4 or technical rejection**	The code submitted does not exist in the current code set. Fix: look up the replacement code and resubmit.
CPT (bundled codes)	**CO-97**	The service is included in another service already billed. The two CPT codes submitted cannot both be paid because one is considered part of the other by the payer's bundling rules (NCCI edits).
CPT (wrong E/M level)	**CO-4 or post-payment audit**	The E/M level billed is not supported by the documentation. Not always a denial up front — often surfaces as a post-payment audit and recoupment request.

CPT (wrong code for service)	**CO-11**	The diagnosis code submitted is inconsistent with the procedure code. Different from CO-4 in that it specifically signals an inconsistency, not just a missing link.
Modifier (missing or wrong)	**CO-4 or CO-97**	Wrong modifier causes the service to appear unbundled when it is legitimately separate, or missing modifier causes a separate service to appear bundled when it is not.
HCPCS (required, not submitted)	**CO-4**	The procedure requires a HCPCS Level II code rather than a CPT code, and CPT was submitted instead. Common in drug administration and DME billing.

> *You do not need to memorize every code. You need to understand the system well enough to know where it broke.*

CHAPTER 3
Reading an Explanation of Benefits Like a Pro

Decode any EOB in under 5 minutes

The Explanation of Benefits is the payer's written response to your claim. It tells you what was paid, what was not paid, and why. It is also one of the most consistently confusing documents in all of healthcare administration — not because the information is not there, but because it is presented in a format designed for efficient payer processing, not for human beings who need to act on it quickly.

Once you understand the anatomy of an EOB, you can read any version of it from any payer in about five minutes. The field names change. The layout changes. The logic underneath never does.

The EOB vs the ERA: Two Formats, One Document

The same information arrives in two formats, and it is worth knowing the difference before we look at the content:

Format	What It Is	When You Use It
EOB (Explanation of Benefits)	A paper or PDF document mailed or posted to the provider's online portal. Human-readable format with patient name, service dates, charges, and reason codes.	When you need to review, print, or discuss a specific claim decision. The EOB is what you send with an appeal.

ERA (Electronic Remittance Advice)	The same payment information transmitted electronically in a standard 835 transaction format. Machine-readable, typically imported directly into the practice management system.	When your billing software auto-posts payments and denials. The ERA drives your denial worklist. The EOB is pulled when you need to take manual action.

> **PRACTICAL TIP:** When you pull an EOB for appeal purposes, always pull the version from the payer's provider portal rather than relying on a printout from your billing software. Software-generated EOB summaries sometimes omit remark codes or truncate reason code descriptions. The payer's own document is the authoritative version.

EOB Anatomy: Every Field Explained

An EOB contains three zones: the header (identifying information about the patient, provider, and payer), the claim detail (line-by-line information about each service), and the summary (totals and patient responsibility). Here is what every key field means and what to do when something looks wrong.

Zone 1: Header Fields

Field	Example Value	What It Means	If Wrong or Missing

Patient Name	`Johnson, Mary A.`	The patient as identified in the payer's system. Must match the name on the insurance card exactly.	Name mismatch = CO-31 or CO-16. Verify registration records. Submit corrected claim with exact name from the insurance card.
Member ID / Subscriber ID	`XYZ123456789`	The unique identifier for this member in the payer's system. This is the most important identifier on the EOB.	Wrong ID = claim submitted to wrong member's policy. Verify ID directly from the insurance card, not from what the patient reports verbally.
Group Number	`GRP-00445`	The employer group associated with the policy. Relevant for COB and for identifying the correct plan when a member has multiple policies.	Wrong group number can cause wrong benefit tier to be applied. Verify from the card.

Claim Number	2024-08-XYZ-001234	The payer's internal reference number for this claim. Always include this on appeals and follow-up calls.	No action if present. If missing from your records: call the payer and request it before submitting an appeal.
Date of Service	08/15/2024	The date the service was rendered. Must match what was billed.	Mismatch = CO-4 or CO-16. Compare to the encounter record and submit corrected claim if different.
Date Received	08/22/2024	The date the payer received the claim. Used to calculate timely filing. Not the same as date of service.	If this date is outside the payer's timely filing window from the date of service: CO-29 denial. You may have a timely filing appeal if you have proof of earlier submission.

Date Processed	09/05/2024	The date the payer adjudicated the claim. Appeal deadlines are usually calculated from this date, not from the date received.	Document this date immediately. Most payers give 30-180 days from this date to file an appeal. Missing the appeal window means losing the right to appeal.

Zone 2: Claim Detail Fields

Field	Example Value	What It Means	If Wrong or Missing
Procedure Code	99214	The CPT or HCPCS code that was adjudicated. Confirm it matches what you submitted.	Mismatch means the payer may have reprocessed your code under a different code (downcoding). This requires an appeal with supporting documentation.

Modifier	-25	Any modifier appended to the procedure code. Confirm it matches your submission.	If the modifier is missing from what was processed, the payer may have stripped it and bundled the service. Appeal with documentation showing the service was distinct.
Diagnosis Code	M54.51	The ICD-10 code submitted with this procedure line. Some EOBs display what was submitted; others display what the payer accepted.	If different from what you submitted: the payer may have mapped your code to a different code during processing. Verify and resubmit if the mapping is incorrect.
Billed Amount	$350.00	What you charged for the service before any contractual adjustments.	This should match your charge master. If it does not, a charge entry error may have occurred.

Allowed Amount	$187.40	The maximum amount the payer will pay for this service under your contract. The contractual adjustment (write-off) is the difference between billed and allowed.	If the allowed amount is lower than expected: check your fee schedule. If there is a discrepancy, contact your payer contract administrator.
Contractual Adjustment	$162.60	The amount written off as a result of your provider contract. Not collectible from the patient.	This should equal Billed minus Allowed. If it does not match your calculations, review your contract for the correct allowed amounts.
Paid to Provider	$149.92	The amount the payer is paying directly to your practice (after deductible, copay, or coinsurance applied).	Post this amount when you receive the check or EFT. Discrepancies between EOB and actual deposit indicate a posting error.
Patient Responsibility	$37.48	The amount the patient owes: deductible, copay, or coinsurance after the payer's payment.	This amount becomes the patient's balance. Do not charge the patient more than this without a contractual basis for doing so.

Adjustment Reason Code	CO-97	The reason for any reduction in payment or denial. This is the most important field for denial management.	See the Adjustment Reason Code section below. Every action you take starts here.
Remark Code	N30	A secondary code providing additional detail about the adjustment. Often more specific and actionable than the reason code alone.	See the Remark Code section below. Always read both reason code AND remark code before deciding how to respond.

Adjustment Reason Codes: The CO/PR/OA System

Every adjustment on an EOB carries a reason code with a two-letter prefix. The prefix tells you who is financially responsible for the adjustment before you read anything else. This is the first thing to look at.

CO	**Contractual Obligation** The payer is reducing payment based on a contractual agreement between the provider and the payer. This is the most common prefix. CO adjustments cannot be billed to the patient — they are write-offs. **Example on EOB:** *CO-45: Charge exceeds fee schedule / maximum allowable. CO-97: Payment included in another service. CO-4: Service inconsistent with diagnosis.*
PR	**Patient Responsibility**

	The adjustment represents an amount the patient is responsible for. This becomes the patient's balance. PR adjustments are billable to the patient. **Example on EOB:** *PR-1: Deductible amount. PR-2: Coinsurance amount. PR-3: Copay amount. These are the three most common PR codes.*

OA	**Other Adjustment** The adjustment does not fit into the CO or PR categories. OA is used for Medicare secondary payer adjustments, coordination of benefits adjustments, and other situations where neither the provider nor the patient is responsible. **Example on EOB:** *OA-23: The impact of prior payer(s) adjudication. Seen on crossover claims where Medicare is primary and Medicaid or a secondary insurer is paying.*

> **THE RULE THAT PREVENTS PATIENT BILLING ERRORS:** Never bill a patient for a CO adjustment. Never. CO adjustments are contractual write-offs. Billing a patient for a CO amount is a contract violation and, in some states, illegal. If a patient is charged for a CO adjustment and pays it, you are required to refund it. PR adjustments — deductible, copay, coinsurance — are the amounts patients legitimately owe.

The 20 Reason Codes You Will See Every Week

These are the adjustment reason codes that appear most frequently in general outpatient physician billing. You do not need to memorize every code in existence. You need to know these twenty well enough to identify the action required without looking them up.

Code	Short Description	What Is Actually Happening	Your First Action

CO-4	**Inconsistent with diagnosis**	The procedure code submitted does not align with the ICD-10 diagnosis code. The clinical link is missing or implausible.	Review the diagnosis and procedure pairing. Determine whether a different ICD-10 code more accurately supports the service, or whether the documentation supports an appeal.
CO-11	**Diagnosis inconsistent with procedure**	Specifically signals a clinical inconsistency between the diagnosis and the procedure, not just a missing link.	Compare the submitted ICD-10 and CPT codes. If the denial is incorrect: gather clinical documentation and appeal. If the code was wrong: submit a corrected claim.
CO-16	**Missing / incorrect information**	A required field on the claim is absent or incorrect. The payer cannot process the claim as submitted.	Check the remark code (often MA130 or N382) for the specific missing field. Correct and resubmit. Common causes: missing NPI, incorrect date of birth, missing referring provider.

CO-18	**Duplicate claim**	A claim for this service has already been submitted and is either pending or paid.	Verify whether the claim was previously submitted. If a previous claim was paid: no action needed unless underpaid. If a previous claim was denied: resubmit with a note that this is a replacement, not a duplicate.
CO-22	**COB / submitted to wrong payer**	This service was covered in whole or in part by another payer. Coordination of benefits applies.	Determine primary and secondary payer. Submit to primary payer first if not done. For secondary: submit with primary EOB attached.
CO-24	**Prior authorization required**	The service required prior authorization that was not obtained, or the authorization number was not included on the claim.	Verify whether an auth was obtained. If yes: resubmit with the auth number on the claim. If no: check whether retro-auth is possible. If not: appeal on medical necessity grounds.

CO-26	**Expenses incurred prior to coverage**	The date of service precedes the patient's effective coverage start date.	Verify the patient's actual effective date with the payer. If the service date is after effective date: appeal with enrollment documentation. If the date is genuinely before coverage: patient is responsible (PR adjustment).
CO-29	**Timely filing**	The claim was submitted after the payer's allowed filing period.	Determine the filing deadline for this payer. If you submitted within the window: gather proof (clearinghouse acknowledgment, prior correspondence) and appeal. If filing genuinely missed: limited recourse.
CO-31	**Patient not eligible**	The patient was not enrolled in or eligible for the plan on the date of service.	Verify eligibility for the specific date of service. If eligible: appeal with documentation. If genuinely ineligible: bill the patient (non-covered service) or write off, depending on your practice policy.

CO-45	**Fee exceeds maximum**	The amount billed exceeds the payer's maximum allowable for the service under your contract.	This is a routine contractual adjustment, not a denial. Post as a write-off. If the allowed amount is lower than your contract specifies: contact your contract administrator.
CO-50	**Non-covered / not medically necessary**	The payer determined the service is not medically necessary based on their coverage criteria.	Obtain the relevant LCD (Local Coverage Determination) or NCD for the service. Appeal with clinical documentation supporting medical necessity. The appeal letter template is in Chapter 11.
CO-57	**No prior authorization obtained**	Authorization was specifically required and was not obtained. (Similar to CO-24 but specifically about authorization absence rather than the claim fields.)	Same process as CO-24. Retro-auth first, then appeal on medical necessity if retro-auth is denied.

CO-97	**Included in another service**	The service billed is considered part of another service already paid or pending payment (bundling).	Identify which code the payer is bundling this service into. Determine whether a modifier (usually -59, -25, or -51) would have separated the service. If applicable: resubmit with the appropriate modifier. If the bundling is incorrect: appeal.
CO-109	**Claim not covered by this payer**	The payer received a claim that should have been sent to a different payer.	Identify the correct payer and resubmit. This often happens when a patient has multiple insurance plans and the primary/secondary sequence is incorrect.
PR-1	**Patient deductible**	This amount is applied to the patient's annual deductible. It is the patient's responsibility.	Post to patient balance and bill the patient. Verify the deductible amount is correct by checking the patient's current deductible accumulation on the payer portal.
PR-2	**Patient coinsurance**	The patient's percentage-based share of the allowed amount. It is the patient's responsibility.	Post to patient balance. Verify the coinsurance percentage matches the patient's plan benefits.

PR-3	**Patient copay**	A fixed dollar amount the patient owes per visit or service. It is the patient's responsibility.	If copay was collected at the time of service: no further action needed. If not collected: post to patient balance and bill.
PR-204	**Not covered by this payer**	The specific service is excluded from coverage under the patient's plan. Patient may be responsible if a waiver (ABN for Medicare) was signed.	Verify whether an ABN or other advance notice was provided. If yes: bill patient. If no: write off.
OA-23	**Impact of prior adjudication**	Adjustment reflects the processing by a prior (primary) payer. Seen on secondary claims.	Verify the primary EOB matches what is reflected here. If the secondary payment calculation appears incorrect, appeal with the primary EOB attached.
OA-999	**Information requested from the patient**	Payer needs information from the patient (not the provider) to complete adjudication. Usually an MSP (Medicare Secondary Payer) questionnaire.	Notify the patient that the payer needs information from them. Some practices have the billing team facilitate this by providing the payer's contact information and the claim reference number.

Remark Codes: The Hidden Second Layer

Remark codes are the detail underneath the adjustment reason code. Every biller knows to look at the reason code. Far fewer consistently check the remark code. This is a significant missed opportunity, because remark codes often contain the specific instruction that turns a vague denial into an actionable fix.

Remark codes use three series:

Series	Prefix	What the Series Covers
MA series	MA1, MA2...	Medicare-specific messages. These provide information about Medicare payment calculations, MSP rules, and remittance messages specific to Medicare claims.
N series	N1, N2...	Provider-level informational messages. These are the most commonly actionable remark codes for commercial payers. N codes often specify exactly what is missing or what needs to be corrected.
M series	M1, M2...	Older Medicare-specific messages, now less commonly used. Some payers still use M-series codes for specific adjustment explanations.

The Remark Codes That Appear Most Often

Code	Short Description	What to Do
MA130	**Additional information needed**	A specific piece of information is required. The code alone does not specify what — call the payer or check the payer's remittance notes for specifics.

N30	**Patient has other insurance**	Coordination of benefits applies. Submit to the other plan and attach the other payer's EOB before submitting to this one as secondary.
N115	**NPI required**	A National Provider Identifier is missing or incorrect on the claim. Identify which NPI is required (rendering, billing, referring) and resubmit.
N130	**Consult your plan documents**	The payer is directing you to the provider manual or contract for details. Usually appears with a denial for a service that is contract-specifically excluded.
N382	**Missing/incomplete/invalid patient identifier**	The patient's member ID or subscriber information is missing or does not match what is on file with the payer.
N432	**Adjustment based on a Recovery Audit finding**	A RAC (Recovery Audit Contractor) has identified this claim for review. This is not a routine denial. Requires documentation submission and may involve repayment.
N517	**Resubmit with itemized bill**	The payer needs an itemized statement of the services provided. Common for hospital claims submitted with a summary UB-04.

N56	**Procedure code not on file**	The CPT code submitted is not recognized under this provider's contract with this payer. Verify the code is covered under your agreement.

ALWAYS READ BOTH CODES: The reason code tells you the category of the problem. The remark code tells you the specific cause. An EOB that shows CO-16 with remark code N115 tells you something completely different from CO-16 with remark code N382. The reason code alone is never enough information to act on confidently.

The 3-Minute EOB Triage

When a denial lands on your desk, you do not have time to read every field before deciding what to do. The following three-minute sequence gets you to a decision on every EOB without missing anything critical.

THE 3-MINUTE EOB TRIAGE SEQUENCE

MINUTE 1: Identify what happened

- Read the adjustment reason code prefix: CO (write-off), PR (patient balance), or OA (other)
- Read the reason code number: what category of problem is this?
- Read the remark code: what specifically is wrong or missing?

MINUTE 2: Classify the action

- APPEAL: Payer made an error, or documentation supports a different decision. The money is recoverable with the right response.
- RESUBMIT: A correctable error on our end (wrong modifier, wrong ID, missing field). Fix and resubmit; no appeal letter needed.
- PATIENT BALANCE: PR adjustment. Post to the patient account and bill the patient.
- WRITE-OFF: CO adjustment that is a legitimate contractual reduction or a genuinely non-covered service with no appeal basis.

MINUTE 3: Decide and route

• APPEAL: Determine which chapter of this book covers this denial type. Prepare the appropriate documentation. Set an appeal deadline in your tickler system.
• RESUBMIT: Correct the specific field identified by the remark code. Resubmit within 48 hours.
• PATIENT BALANCE: Post and generate the patient statement.
• WRITE-OFF: Post the adjustment and close the claim.

When the EOB Does Not Give You Enough Information

Some denials arrive with reason codes that are technically accurate but practically useless. CO-16 tells you something is missing but not what. CO-4 tells you the service is inconsistent with the diagnosis but not which diagnosis or why. In these cases, there are three additional sources of information:

- Call the payer's provider services line: have the claim number, patient name, member ID, and date of service ready before you call. Ask specifically: 'What information is missing from this claim?' or 'Which diagnosis code do you need to support this procedure?' Document the name of the representative, the date and time of the call, and exactly what they tell you.
- Check the payer's online portal: most major commercial payers now provide denial reason detail in their provider portal that exceeds what appears on the paper or PDF EOB. Log in and pull up the claim for additional notes.
- Request the clinical policy: if the denial is for medical necessity, request the specific coverage policy (LCD, NCD, or commercial medical policy) the payer applied. You are entitled to know which policy governs the denial and what criteria must be met for the service to be covered. This information is the foundation of a successful medical necessity appeal.

Every denial contains a message. The reason code is the headline. The remark code is the story. Read both before you decide what to do next.

CHAPTER 4 · PART 2: THE 12 DENIAL TYPES DECODED

Eligibility and Coverage Denials

CO-4, CO-31 — denied before the claim even starts

These denials are the most preventable category in all of medical billing. They happen before the service is coded, before the claim is built, before anyone has looked at what was documented in the chart. They happen at the front door — at scheduling, at check-in, at the moment someone typed the wrong insurance card into the system or forgot to check whether coverage was still active.

That is what makes them so frustrating. By the time a CO-4 or CO-31 denial arrives, the appointment has happened, the physician has seen the patient, and the service has been rendered. The money may never come back. But the process that caused it is still running, producing the same denial on the same type of patient every week.

This chapter gives you the fix for the denials already in your queue, and the workflow change that stops them from arriving.

Understanding the Two Denial Types

Eligibility and coverage denials are related but not identical. The distinction matters because the fix is different for each.

Code	What It Means	Root Cause

CO-31	Patient not eligible on the date of service. The patient did not have active coverage with this payer at the time the service was provided.	(1) Coverage lapsed or was terminated between the last eligibility verification and the date of service. (2) The patient provided the wrong insurance information. (3) Eligibility was not verified at all before the visit.
CO-4	Service not covered by the patient's plan. The patient has active coverage, but the specific service billed is excluded from their benefit package.	(1) The service is a plan exclusion (e.g., cosmetic procedures, certain alternative therapies). (2) The service requires authorization that was not obtained. (3) The diagnosis submitted does not support coverage of the procedure under this plan's medical policies.
CO-26	Date of service precedes the patient's coverage effective date. The patient was not yet enrolled in the plan when the service was rendered.	(1) New employee or new plan year — coverage started after the appointment date. (2) Patient enrolled in new plan but provided old insurance card. (3) Retroactive termination by prior plan overlaps with new plan effective date.
CO-27	Expenses incurred after coverage terminated. The patient's coverage ended before the date of service.	(1) Job change, divorce, or aging off a parent's plan. (2) Non-payment of premium resulting in retroactive termination. (3) Patient not aware that coverage ended.

CO-31: Patient Not Eligible

CO-31	Patient Not Eligible	**Frequency:** Very High — top 5 denial category	**Appeal success:** Moderate: 40-60% if proof of eligibility exists

Why This Happens More Than It Should

The most common assumption in practices that see high CO-31 rates: 'We verified insurance.' The problem is what 'verified insurance' actually means in most workflows. If verification means calling the payer's automated IVR line once at scheduling and not again, the practice is checking eligibility at the wrong moment and never catching the changes that happen between scheduling and the date of service.

Coverage changes happen constantly. Employers switch plans on January 1. Employees lose jobs. Cobra coverage lapses. Spouses remove a partner from their plan during divorce proceedings. A patient who was eligible on Monday may not be eligible on Friday. And many patients do not know their coverage has changed until after the service — sometimes not until they receive a bill.

The Five Most Common CO-31 Scenarios

Scenario	What Actually Happened and What to Do
Retroactive termination	The payer terminates coverage effective a past date, meaning coverage that appeared active at the time of the visit was retroactively cancelled. This is the most difficult CO-31 scenario because eligibility verification would have shown the patient as covered. Options: (1) Appeal with proof of eligibility verification at time of service. (2) Bill the patient as self-pay if unable to recover from payer. (3) Request an itemized explanation from the payer of the retroactive termination date.
Wrong insurance on file	The patient provided insurance information that is no longer active — an old employer plan, an expired COBRA policy, or a plan they switched away from. At the time of service, no one asked to see the physical insurance card. Fix: always scan or photograph both sides of the insurance card at every visit, not just the first visit.

COB sequence incorrect	The patient has two insurance plans and the claim was sent to the wrong one as primary, or the secondary was billed without the primary EOB. The primary payer returns CO-31 because this service should have been processed by the other plan first. Fix: verify COB status and determine correct primary/secondary sequence before submitting.
New plan year, same patient	The patient's employer changed plans on January 1 (or another plan year start date) and the new insurance information was not collected. The old plan card on file generates CO-31. Fix: collect and verify new insurance at the first visit of each calendar year, regardless of whether the patient reports any changes.
Aged off parent's plan	A young adult patient aged off a parent's insurance at age 26 and either did not obtain new coverage or obtained new coverage but did not update their information with the practice. Fix: flag patients approaching age 26 for proactive re-verification.

FIX IT: What to do with this denial today

1. Pull the original eligibility verification you ran for this patient on the date of service. If you ran it and it showed active coverage, attach that verification result to your appeal. Many payers will overturn CO-31 denials when you can document that the patient appeared eligible at the time of service.

2. If you did not verify eligibility before the visit: call the payer's provider services line and ask for the specific date coverage terminated. This tells you whether the termination was retroactive (appealable) or the patient genuinely had no coverage (explore patient self-pay options).

3. Contact the patient and inform them of the denial. Ask them to contact their HR department or insurance carrier to verify whether coverage was active. Sometimes the patient can resolve a retroactive termination issue with their own employer.

4. If the appeal is denied: bill the patient. A CO-31 denial does not eliminate patient responsibility. Depending on your state and your payer contract, you may be able to collect from the patient as self-pay.

PREVENT IT: What to change so it stops happening

1. Verify eligibility no earlier than 24-48 hours before the appointment, not at scheduling. Use real-time eligibility (270/271 transactions) through your clearinghouse or practice management system for the most current response.
2. Verify eligibility again on the morning of the appointment for any patient scheduled for a service with a significant copay or deductible exposure.
3. At check-in: always ask the patient 'Has your insurance changed since your last visit?' and scan the physical insurance card even if the answer is no. Cards change. People forget.
4. Build a report in your practice management system to flag patients whose last eligibility verification is more than 30 days old. Run this report weekly and re-verify before appointments.
5. For annual re-enrollments (common January 1 for employer plans): contact your patient panel in November to update insurance information proactively before the new plan year begins.

CO-4: Service Not Covered

CO-4	**Service Not Covered / Inconsistent With Diagnosis**	**Frequency:** Very High — #1 or #2 denial in most practices	**Appeal success:** Low to Moderate: depends on whether a coding fix or appeal is needed

CO-4 is the most commonly used denial code in the system, and it covers two distinct problems that require different responses:

CO-4 Type	What Is Happening

Type A: Diagnosis does not support the procedure	The ICD-10 code submitted does not clinically justify the CPT code billed. The payer's automated editing system checks whether the diagnosis is one that their coverage policies recognize as a valid reason to perform the procedure. If not: CO-4.
Type B: Service excluded from the patient's plan	The service is simply not covered under this patient's benefit package — regardless of the diagnosis. Common exclusions: cosmetic procedures, certain dental services, infertility treatments, weight loss surgery, specific alternative therapies.

HOW TO TELL WHICH TYPE YOU HAVE: Type A (coding/linking problem) will often accompany a remark code like N386 or refer to a specific diagnosis-procedure inconsistency. Type B (plan exclusion) will typically state the service is 'not a benefit of the patient's plan' or reference the patient's benefit package. Calling the payer and asking 'Is this service excluded from this patient's plan, or is there a coverage policy I can reference?' will clarify which type you are dealing with.

CO-4 Type A: Fixing the Diagnosis-Procedure Link

This is the most fixable version of CO-4, and the most common. The diagnosis submitted was either too non-specific, incorrectly linked to the procedure, or not aligned with the payer's coverage criteria for that procedure.

- Step 1: Pull the clinical documentation. Read what the physician actually documented — the chief complaint, the assessment, and the plan. The correct ICD-10 code must come from what is documented, not from what you think should be there.
- Step 2: Identify whether a more specific ICD-10 code exists that better represents the documented condition and more clearly supports the procedure. Use a current ICD-10-CM codebook or encoder.
- Step 3: Check the payer's medical policy or LCD (Local Coverage Determination) for this procedure. The LCD

specifies exactly which ICD-10 codes the payer considers as valid coverage criteria for the service.

- Step 4: If a more appropriate code exists AND the documentation supports it: submit a corrected claim with the revised ICD-10 code. This is a resubmission, not an appeal.
- Step 5: If the documentation genuinely does not support a diagnosis that meets the payer's coverage criteria: the denial may be valid. Discuss with the physician whether the documentation accurately reflects what was clinically present.

CO-4 Type B: When the Service Is Truly Excluded

When a service is excluded from the patient's benefit package, the appeal options are limited. However, there are still steps worth taking before writing off the claim:

- Verify the exclusion: call the payer and ask them to cite the specific plan document or benefit exclusion that applies to this service. Not all CO-4 denials labeled as exclusions are correctly coded. Some are actually Type A denials labeled as exclusions by the automated system.
- Check for a medical necessity override: some plans exclude a service in general but cover it when specific medical criteria are met. The payer's medical policy will specify whether an exception is available.
- Issue an Advance Beneficiary Notice (ABN) for Medicare patients: if the service is non-covered by Medicare and you knew or expected it would not be covered before the service was rendered, an ABN allows you to collect from the patient instead. Without the ABN, you cannot bill the Medicare patient for the non-covered service.
- Bill the patient: for non-Medicare patients, if the service is excluded from their benefit package and you did not have a contractual obligation to provide it for free, the patient may be responsible. Review your payer contract for balance billing restrictions.

FIX IT: What to do with this denial today

1. Determine whether this is a Type A (linking) or Type B (exclusion) denial using the method above.

2. For Type A: pull documentation, identify the correct ICD-10 code, check the payer's LCD, and submit a corrected claim if a valid link exists.

3. For Type B: verify the exclusion, check for a medical necessity override path, and determine patient billing options based on your contract and any pre-service ABN or waiver.

4. Document all steps taken and the outcome in the claim notes field of your practice management system.

PREVENT IT: What to change so it stops happening

1. Run pre-submission claim edits: most practice management systems and clearinghouses offer code-pair editing (NCCI edits) and payer-specific edits that flag diagnosis-procedure inconsistencies before the claim goes out. Enable these edits and review every flagged claim before submission.

2. For high-volume procedures with specific coverage criteria (imaging, injections, preventive screenings): build an ICD-10 diagnosis reference list for each CPT code that your practice uses frequently. Confirm the correct diagnosis is linked before coding.

3. For new patients or patients receiving a service for the first time: verify coverage for that specific service type before the appointment. Ask the payer: 'Is CPT [code] covered under this patient's plan, and if so, what diagnosis requirements apply?'

4. Train front desk to collect and record the patient's plan type (HMO, PPO, HDHP) at registration. Plan type affects coverage exclusions and referral requirements in ways that eligibility verification alone does not capture.

The Eligibility Verification Checklist

The single most effective tool for reducing eligibility and coverage denials is a standardized eligibility verification process. The following checklist covers every field that matters. Run this check for every patient before every appointment.

ELIGIBILITY VERIFICATION CHECKLIST — 8 FIELDS TO CONFIRM

1. Coverage status: Is coverage active as of today's date? Not the scheduling date — today.

2. Effective and termination dates: When did coverage start? Does it have an end date? Is a COBRA or continuation period involved?

3. Plan type: HMO (requires referral?), PPO (any network restrictions?), HDHP (high deductible — what is the remaining deductible balance?), Medicare Advantage (different from traditional Medicare).

4. Covered services and exclusions: For any non-routine or specialized service scheduled: is that specific service type covered under this plan?

5. Authorization requirements: Does this service type require prior authorization under this plan? Does this specialty require a referral from a PCP?

6. Deductible and out-of-pocket: What is the patient's remaining deductible? Has the out-of-pocket maximum been reached? This affects patient communication, not billing, but it prevents balance disputes.

7. Coordination of benefits: Does the patient have any other insurance? Which is primary? Never assume a patient has only one plan.

8. Network status: Is your practice in-network for this specific plan? (Not just the payer — the specific plan. Many payers have multiple networks with different participating providers.)

When to Verify vs When to Trust the System

Many practice management systems offer automated real-time eligibility verification through a 270/271 transaction. This is faster than a manual call and is accurate at the moment the request is submitted. However, 270/271 responses have two important limitations:

- They confirm what the payer knows at the moment of the request, not what will be true on the date of service. A plan that is active today may be terminated tomorrow through an employer action. For services scheduled more than a week in advance: reverify within 48 hours of the appointment.

- They do not always capture service-specific coverage details. The 270/271 response may confirm active coverage but will not always specify whether a particular procedure type is covered under the patient's exact plan. For high-cost or specialty services: supplement the automated check with a coverage verification call for that specific service.

DOCUMENT EVERY VERIFICATION: For every eligibility verification you perform, document the date and time of verification, the method used (real-time electronic, phone call, portal), the name or ID of the payer representative if a call was made, and the coverage status confirmed. This documentation is your evidence in a CO-31 appeal and your protection in a payer audit. A claim that was denied because coverage was retroactively terminated can be appealed successfully when you have documented proof that coverage appeared active at the time you verified.

Before and After: The Workflow Change That Works

The following comparison shows the difference between the verification workflow that produces high CO-31 and CO-4 rates and the workflow that eliminates most of them. The changes are not expensive or technically complex. They require consistency.

Workflow That Produces Denials	Workflow That Prevents Denials
Eligibility verified once at scheduling, 1-2 weeks before the appointment	Eligibility verified within 48 hours of the appointment date
Patient verbally confirms 'same insurance' — not re-verified	Insurance card scanned at every visit, even for established patients

No service-specific coverage check for specialty or non-routine services	Coverage call made for any service with significant CO-4 risk (imaging, injections, procedures)
COB not checked — assumed single payer	COB question asked at every visit: 'Do you have any other insurance?'
Verification not documented — no evidence available for appeal	Verification documented in the patient record: date, method, result
New plan year not proactively addressed	Patient contact campaign in November to collect new plan-year insurance information
Front desk not trained on reading the plan type from the insurance card	Front desk training on HMO vs PPO vs HDHP and referral/auth implications of each

> *Eligibility denials are not a billing problem. They are a front-desk process problem that billing pays for.*

CHAPTER 5 · PART 2: THE 12 DENIAL TYPES DECODED

Duplicate Claim Denials

CO-97, CO-18 — the claim you already submitted

Duplicate claim denials feel like bureaucratic punishment. You submitted the claim. The payer did not pay it or did not respond within a reasonable timeframe. You submitted it again. Now the payer denies both as duplicates.

The frustrating part is that duplicate denials can come from two entirely different situations: a genuinely resubmitted claim (where the first submission was lost or ignored) and a bundled service that the payer is treating as already included in another payment. Both arrive with similar-looking denial codes. They require completely different responses.

This chapter separates them clearly and gives you the response for each.

CO-18 vs CO-97: Not the Same Problem

Before you respond to any duplicate denial, identify which code you are looking at. The action is different for each.

Code	What It Technically Says	What Is Actually Happening

CO-18	Exact duplicate claim or service	The payer has already received and either processed or is currently processing an identical claim — same patient, same date of service, same procedure code, same provider. A second submission for the same service arrived.
CO-97	Payment included in allowance for another service	The service billed is bundled into another procedure already paid or pending payment. This is a bundling denial, not a true duplicate. The payer is saying: we already compensated for this as part of something else.

THE CRITICAL DISTINCTION: CO-18 means the payer saw this exact claim twice. CO-97 means the payer believes this service is already included in another payment. Resubmitting a CO-97 without a modifier change will result in another CO-97. Appealing a CO-18 without proof of original submission will fail. Knowing which one you have determines every subsequent step.

CO-18: True Duplicate Claim

CO-18	Exact Duplicate Claim	**Frequency:** Moderate — often triggered by biller resubmission during follow-up	**Appeal rate:** High: 70-80% when original submission is documented

The Three Scenarios That Produce CO-18

Scenario	What Happened and What to Do

Biller resubmitted during follow-up, first claim was already in process	The original claim was submitted on time and is pending in the payer's system. The biller, not seeing a response after 30 days, resubmitted. The payer receives the second claim while the first is still pending and denies the second as a duplicate. Fix: always check claim status through the payer portal or clearinghouse tracking before resubmitting. If a claim is pending, wait. If a claim is truly lost, use a replacement claim (billing frequency code 7), not a new submission.
Clearinghouse submitted the claim twice	Clearinghouse transmission errors can occasionally submit a claim more than once. This is rare with modern clearinghouses but still occurs. Fix: contact your clearinghouse and request the transmission log for the date in question. The clearinghouse should resolve the duplicate and confirm the original submission was received. Document the clearinghouse confirmation for your appeal.
Two billers submitted the same claim independently	In practices with multiple billing staff or outsourced billing alongside in-house staff, the same claim can be submitted by two people working from different worklists. Fix: trace both submissions in your practice management system. Identify which was submitted first. The first submission is the legitimate one. Write off the duplicate denial and monitor the first submission for payment.

How to Investigate a CO-18 Before Responding

- Step 1: Pull both claim submissions from your practice management system. Compare the submission dates, the claim numbers, and the clearinghouse acknowledgment records for each.
- Step 2: Log into the payer's provider portal and look up the claim by patient name, date of service, and procedure code. Determine the status of the original claim. If the original is pending: wait for it to process. If the original was paid: no further action needed, write off the duplicate denial. If the

original was denied for a different reason: that is the claim that needs attention.

- Step 3: If the original claim cannot be located in the payer's system and you have clearinghouse acknowledgment that it was transmitted: you have evidence for a timely filing protection appeal on the duplicate.

FIX IT: What to do with this denial today

1. Determine the status of the original claim before doing anything else. Log into the payer portal using the original claim number.

2. If the original is pending: write a note in your system and wait. Do not resubmit again. Check status again in 15 days.

3. If the original was paid: post the payment to the correct claim. The CO-18 denial on the second submission is correct — write it off.

4. If the original was denied for a different reason: work the original denial. The CO-18 duplicate can be written off once the original is resolved.

5. If the original cannot be found in the payer system but you have clearinghouse proof of submission: appeal the CO-18 with the clearinghouse acknowledgment record attached as evidence.

PREVENT IT: What to change so it stops happening

1. Check claim status in the payer portal or clearinghouse tracking before any resubmission. The rule: never resubmit without confirming the original is not already in process.

2. Establish a follow-up workflow with a defined waiting period by payer type: Medicare (30 days), commercial payers (30-45 days), Medicaid (45-60 days). Only initiate resubmission inquiry after the payer's standard processing time has passed.

3. Use replacement claims (billing frequency type code 7) rather than new submissions when correcting a pending claim. A replacement claim links to the original and reduces duplicate risk.

4. In practices with multiple billing staff: assign specific date-of-service ranges or provider assignments to each biller so the same claim cannot be worked by two people simultaneously.

CO-97: Bundling Denial (Payment Already Included)

CO-97	Payment Included in Another Service	**Frequency:** High — among the most common denial codes	**Appeal rate:** Moderate: 50-60% with correct modifier and documentation

CO-97 is one of the most misunderstood denial codes in medical billing, because the name suggests a duplicate but the reality is bundling. The payer is not saying you submitted the claim twice. The payer is saying: the service you billed is considered part of another service we already paid, so we are not paying for it separately.

The rules governing what is and is not bundled come from the National Correct Coding Initiative (NCCI), maintained by CMS. NCCI edits define code pairs that cannot be billed together without a modifier that documents a specific exception. Commercial payers also have their own bundling rules in addition to NCCI.

The Three Types of CO-97 Bundling

Bundling Type	What the Payer Is Saying	Can a Modifier Fix It?
NCCI Comprehensive/ Component bundling	Code A includes Code B by definition. Example: a surgical procedure code includes the closure of the incision — billing both produces CO-97. The component code is always included in the comprehensive code.	Sometimes. If the component service was genuinely performed separately from the comprehensive service (different body site, different session), modifier -59 or an X-modifier may apply.

Global surgical package bundling	A service billed within the global period (0, 10, or 90 days post-surgery) is considered part of the surgical package. Example: billing an office visit 5 days after minor surgery without a modifier.	Yes, with the correct modifier: -24 (E/M unrelated to surgery), -79 (unrelated procedure), or -58 (staged procedure). The service must be genuinely unrelated to or specifically planned separately from the original procedure.
Mutually exclusive code pairs	Two codes that by definition cannot both be performed at the same time on the same patient. NCCI identifies these as column 1/column 2 pairs where neither can ever be billed with the other, even with a modifier.	No. Mutually exclusive edits with a 0 modifier indicator cannot be overridden. If you see this denial on a code pair with a 0 indicator, the bundling is absolute.

NCCI: What It Is and How to Use It

The National Correct Coding Initiative edit tables are publicly available on the CMS website at no cost. They list every code pair that is subject to a bundling edit and indicate whether the edit can be overridden with a modifier. You should bookmark this resource and check it before billing any combination of codes that might be subject to bundling.

- Modifier indicator 0: the edit cannot be overridden by any modifier. Do not bill these codes together under any circumstances.
- Modifier indicator 1: the edit can be overridden with an appropriate modifier (-25, -59, -91, or X-modifiers) when the clinical circumstances justify separate billing. Documentation must support the modifier.

HOW TO LOOK UP AN NCCI EDIT: Go to cms.gov and search 'NCCI edit files.' Download the current quarter's Practitioner PTP (Procedure-to-Procedure) edit table. Open in Excel. Use Ctrl+F to search for the column 1 or column 2 code. The table will show the code pair, the effective date, the deletion date (if any), and the modifier indicator (0 or 1). Update your reference file quarterly when CMS releases new edits.

The Modifier Question: When Can You Override the Bundle?

When a CO-97 denial arrives and the NCCI modifier indicator is 1 (meaning the edit can be overridden), the next question is whether the clinical circumstances actually justify a separate billing — and whether the modifier that would separate it was correctly applied.

Modifier	When It Justifies Separate Billing	Documentation Required
-25	A significant, separately identifiable E/M service was performed on the same day as a procedure by the same physician.	The note must document the E/M service as distinct from the pre-procedure assessment. The chief complaint, history, examination, and medical decision making for the E/M should be separately identifiable from the procedure note.
-59	The procedure or service was distinct from other services on the same day: different anatomic site, different session, or separate injury.	Documentation must clearly establish the distinctness: separate location, separate incision, separate organ, or separate patient encounter. 'Routine' use of -59 to override bundles is a compliance risk.
-91	The same lab test was repeated on the same day to obtain subsequent results.	The clinical reason for the repeat test must be documented. Cannot be used for repeat tests due to equipment failure or specimen quality issues.

XE, XS, XP, XU	CMS-specific modifiers that provide more granular justification for separate billing than -59 alone.	XE: separate encounter. XS: separate structure (different anatomical site). XP: separate practitioner. XU: unusual non-overlapping service. Use the most specific X-modifier before defaulting to -59.

FIX IT: What to do with this denial today

1. Look up the denied code pair in the NCCI edit table. Identify the modifier indicator: 0 (cannot override) or 1 (can override with documentation).

2. If modifier indicator is 0: the bundling is absolute. Write off the column 2 code. Do not appeal.

3. If modifier indicator is 1: review the original claim to determine whether a modifier was present. If no modifier was submitted: determine whether the clinical circumstances justify separate billing. If yes, resubmit with the appropriate modifier (-25, -59, XE, XS, XP, or XU).

4. If a modifier was submitted but still denied: review the documentation to confirm it supports the modifier. If documentation is sufficient, appeal with a copy of the relevant portions of the medical record and a written explanation of why the services were separately identifiable.

5. For global surgical package CO-97s: identify the post-operative period (0, 10, or 90 days), determine the correct modifier for the situation (-24, -58, -79), and resubmit with the modifier and documentation of the unrelated condition.

PREVENT IT: What to change so it stops happening

1. Enable NCCI edits in your practice management system or clearinghouse. Most systems allow you to run claims through NCCI logic before submission. Claims that trigger a bundle edit are flagged for review before they go out.

2. Build a modifier decision tree for your most-used code pairs. For any CPT code that your practice bills frequently alongside other codes (E/M plus procedure, multiple procedures in one session): create a reference card that specifies when each modifier applies and what documentation is required.

3. Conduct a monthly bundling audit: pull 10 randomly selected claims that included multiple procedure codes and verify that each code combination was appropriate and correctly modified.

4. Train coders and billers on the global surgical package rules for the procedures your practice performs. Know the global period (0, 10, or 90 days) for every surgical code in your charge master.
5. When adding a new procedure to your practice's services: look up its NCCI edit pairs before billing it the first time. Build the modifier rules into your charge entry process from day one.

Clearinghouse Tracking: Know Before the Denial Arrives

The most effective tool for avoiding both CO-18 and CO-97 denials is clearinghouse tracking visibility. Most practices submit claims and then wait for a response. Practices with low duplicate denial rates actively monitor claim status through the clearinghouse and payer portals from the moment of submission.

Clearinghouse Status	What It Means and What to Do
Acknowledged / Accepted	The clearinghouse received the claim and forwarded it to the payer. The claim is in the payer's queue. No action needed yet. Begin follow-up if no response within the payer's standard processing window (typically 30 days for commercial, 14 days for Medicare).
Rejected by clearinghouse	The claim failed a clearinghouse technical edit (missing NPI, wrong format, invalid code). This is a rejection, not a denial. Fix the identified error and resubmit immediately. The clock is running on timely filing.
Pending at payer	The payer has received the claim and is processing it. Do not resubmit. Resubmitting a pending claim generates a CO-18 duplicate denial.
Denied by payer	The claim was adjudicated and denied. Pull the EOB to identify the reason code and begin the appropriate response workflow.

No status / Not found	The claim cannot be located in the clearinghouse or payer system. This is the situation that warrants resubmission — but first confirm the original submission date and clearinghouse record before resending.

> **THE FOLLOW-UP CALENDAR:** Build a follow-up tickler in your practice management system for every claim submitted. Standard follow-up windows: Medicare = 30 days from submission. Commercial = 30-45 days. Medicaid = 45-60 days (varies by state). When the tickler fires, check status in the payer portal before taking any action. If the claim is pending: reset the tickler for another 15 days. If the claim is not found: initiate a replacement claim with documentation of original submission. Never resubmit without checking status first.

Bundling Basics: The 20-Minute Reference

You do not need to memorize every NCCI edit pair. You need to understand the underlying logic of bundling so you can recognize a CO-97 situation before the claim goes out. The following table covers the bundling concepts that produce the most CO-97 denials in outpatient physician billing.

Bundling Concept	Common Example	Correct Approach
Incision and closure	Billing a laceration repair CPT code AND a separate closure code for the same wound	The repair code already includes closure. Do not bill a separate closure code. One code covers the complete repair.
Surgical approach and procedure	Billing the approach (e.g., laparoscopy) separately from the procedure performed through it	The approach is included in the surgical procedure code. Bill only the procedure code.

E/M same day as minor procedure	Billing an office visit (99213-99215) on the same day as a minor procedure (0-day global) without modifier -25	Append -25 to the E/M only if the E/M was significant and separately identifiable from the pre-procedure assessment. The documentation must support it.
Lab panel and component tests	Billing a lab panel code (e.g., 80050 for a general health panel) AND the individual component tests (glucose, CBC, etc.) separately	When a panel code exists and the components were all performed, bill the panel code only. Billing the panel and the components produces CO-97 on the components.
Bilateral procedures	Billing the same unilateral procedure code twice for left and right sides	Most bilateral procedures are handled with modifier -50 (bilateral) on a single procedure code line, not by submitting the code twice. Submitting twice generates CO-18 or CO-97 depending on the payer.
Supervision and interpretation	Billing both a supervision code and a separate interpretation code for the same imaging service when the physician performed only one component	If the physician supervised but did not interpret: bill the supervision component only. If only interpreted: bill the interpretation with modifier -26. If both: bill the global code without a modifier.

> *CO-18 is a process problem. CO-97 is a coding problem. The solution to each lives in a completely different part of your workflow.*

CHAPTER 6 · PART 2: THE 12 DENIAL TYPES DECODED

Prior Authorization Denials

Denied for no auth, wrong auth, or expired auth

Prior authorization is the process by which a payer reviews a planned service before it is rendered and decides whether it will cover the cost. When it works, it gives the practice advance certainty of payment. When it fails — when no authorization was obtained, or the wrong service was authorized, or the authorization expired before the service occurred — the resulting denial is among the most expensive in medical billing because it applies to high-cost services: surgeries, specialty referrals, advanced imaging, infusions, and inpatient admissions.

The AMA's annual prior authorization survey consistently finds that prior auth requirements have increased significantly over the past decade, with physicians and their staff spending an average of nearly two full business days per week on prior authorization tasks. Despite that investment, auth-related denials remain stubbornly common because the authorization process requires precision — the right service, the right code, the right provider, the right timeframe — and any single mismatch produces a denial.

This chapter covers all three auth denial types, the retro-auth path when available, and the tracking system that prevents most of them.

The Three Types of Prior Auth Denials

Type	Denial Reason	Root Cause

Type 1	**No authorization obtained. The service required prior auth and none was requested before the service was rendered.**	(1) Staff did not know this service required auth for this payer. (2) Auth was requested but not received before the appointment proceeded. (3) The service was added or changed at the time of the encounter without checking auth requirements.
Type 2	**Authorization mismatch. An authorization was obtained, but the service billed does not match what was authorized — different CPT code, different provider, different facility, or different date range.**	(1) The procedure changed between the auth request and the service date. (2) A covering provider performed the service instead of the authorized provider. (3) The authorization was obtained using a preliminary diagnosis or code that changed after further evaluation.
Type 3	**Authorization expired. An authorization was obtained but the service was not rendered within the authorized date range.**	(1) Surgery or procedure was rescheduled beyond the auth end date without obtaining a new authorization. (2) Authorization was obtained far in advance and expired before the patient's insurance approved the final schedule. (3) No one tracked the expiration date.

Type 1: No Authorization Obtained

CO-24 /CO-57	No Prior Authorization	**Frequency:** High — among the most expensive denial categories by dollar value	**Appeal rate:** Low without retro-auth. Moderate with retro-auth: 30-50%

The Retro-Authorization Path

When a service was rendered without authorization and the claim is denied, the first question is whether the payer allows retroactive authorization — also called retro-auth or post-service auth. Retro-auth is a process by which the payer reviews the medical necessity of the service after it was already performed and, if approved, treats the authorization as if it had been obtained in advance.

Not every payer allows retro-auth, and those that do have strict timeframes — typically 24 to 72 hours for emergent services and 5 to 30 business days for non-emergent services. The window is short. This is the first call to make when a no-auth denial arrives.

Service Type	Retro-Auth Availability and Approach
Emergency or urgent service	Most payers are required by state and federal law to cover emergency services regardless of prior authorization. If the service was genuinely emergent, the denial should be appealed on that basis with clinical documentation supporting the emergent nature. The auth requirement does not apply to true emergencies.
Non-emergent service, payer allows retro-auth	Call the payer's prior auth department immediately upon receiving the denial. Request a retro-auth review. Provide: (1) the patient's member ID, (2) the service date and CPT code, (3) the rendering provider's NPI, and (4) clinical documentation supporting medical necessity. A retro-auth approval converts the claim denial into a payable claim upon resubmission with the auth number.
Non-emergent service, payer does not allow retro-auth	If retro-auth is not available and the service was not emergent: appeal on medical necessity grounds with full clinical documentation. The appeal argues that the service met the payer's coverage criteria even though auth was not obtained. Success rate is low unless the payer's own coverage policy clearly supports the service.

Non-emergent service, patient was informed in advance	If the patient was informed before the service that authorization may be required or that the claim may not be covered, and a financial waiver or ABN was signed, bill the patient for the service. This does not apply to Medicare Advantage without a proper ABN process.

FIX IT: What to do with this denial today

1. Identify the service type: emergent or non-emergent. If emergent, appeal immediately on emergency services grounds with supporting clinical documentation. Do not request retro-auth for emergencies — appeal directly.

2. If non-emergent: call the payer's prior auth department within 24 hours of receiving the denial and ask specifically: 'Does this payer allow retroactive authorization for this service type, and what is the submission window?' Document the representative's name, date, and response.

3. If retro-auth is available: submit the retro-auth request with clinical documentation supporting medical necessity. Use the same format as a standard auth request (see Section 6.3). Follow up within 5 business days.

4. If retro-auth is approved: resubmit the claim with the retro-auth number in the authorization field. Note on the claim that this is a resubmission following retro-auth approval.

5. If retro-auth is denied: file a formal appeal on medical necessity grounds. The appeal letter should cite the payer's own coverage policy for this service and document why the clinical criteria were met.

PREVENT IT: What to change so it stops happening

1. Build a payer-specific auth requirement matrix: a simple spreadsheet listing every payer your practice bills, the services that require auth for each payer, and the auth request lead time required. Update it whenever a payer sends a notification of coverage change.

2. Assign auth responsibility clearly: one person or team owns the auth process from request through confirmation. When auth responsibility is shared without clear ownership, things fall through the cracks.

3. Never schedule a service that requires auth without a confirmed auth number in hand. Pending or in-process auth is not the same as approved auth. The appointment is not confirmed until the auth is confirmed.
4. Check auth requirements at the point of scheduling, not the day before the appointment. For services with 5-to-10-business-day auth turnaround: start the request the moment the appointment is scheduled.
5. Train clinical staff to alert the billing team immediately when the planned service changes at the time of the encounter. A different procedure than what was scheduled may require a different auth.

Type 2: Authorization Mismatch

CO-24	**Authorization Obtained But Does Not Match Service**	**Frequency:** Moderate — common in surgical and specialty practices	**Appeal rate:** Moderate to High: 55-70% when mismatch is minor and documented

An auth mismatch denial occurs when an authorization exists but the service rendered does not match the authorization on one or more key fields. The payer compares what was authorized against what was billed and finds a discrepancy.

Mismatch Type	What Happened	Response
CPT code mismatch	The procedure code billed is different from the procedure code on the authorization. Example: auth obtained for 27447 (total knee arthroplasty), but 27446 (unicompartmental knee replacement) was performed.	If the procedure genuinely changed: request a new or amended authorization for the actual procedure performed. Appeal with operative notes documenting the change and its clinical basis.

Provider mismatch	The authorization was issued for Provider A, but the service was rendered by Provider B (a covering physician, a different group member, or a locum tenens provider).	Call the payer and request that the auth be transferred to the rendering provider's NPI. Many payers allow this with a simple phone request when providers are in the same group. Document the transfer confirmation.
Facility mismatch	The authorization was for Facility A but the service was performed at Facility B.	If the facility change was planned: the auth should have been updated. Contact the payer, explain the facility change, and request an amended auth. If the change was unplanned (e.g., emergency room diversion): appeal on that basis with documentation.
Date range mismatch	The service was rendered outside the authorized date range, either before the start date or after the end date.	If the service date falls within a reasonable extension: call the payer and request an extension of the auth dates. Many payers will extend by phone if the auth was otherwise valid. If the auth has fully expired: see Type 3 below.

Diagnosis code mismatch	The ICD-10 code on the claim differs from the ICD-10 code used in the auth request. Common when the working diagnosis at auth time differs from the confirmed diagnosis at service time.	If the diagnosis genuinely changed and the new diagnosis still meets coverage criteria: appeal with clinical documentation explaining the diagnostic evolution. If the correct diagnosis should have been on the auth: request an amended auth.

FIX IT: What to do with this denial today

1. Pull the original authorization confirmation and compare it field by field against what was billed: CPT code, rendering provider NPI, facility NPI, authorized dates, and diagnosis code.

2. Identify the specific mismatch. Call the payer's prior auth department and explain the discrepancy. Ask whether an amended authorization can be issued retroactively to cover the service as rendered.

3. If the payer will issue an amended auth: obtain the new auth number, document the call (representative name, date, time), and resubmit the claim with the corrected authorization number.

4. If the payer will not issue an amended auth: appeal the denial with supporting documentation — operative report, clinical notes, and a written explanation of why the service rendered was clinically equivalent to or consistent with what was authorized.

5. Document the outcome in your auth tracking log regardless of result.

PREVENT IT: What to change so it stops happening

1. At the point of auth confirmation: enter the authorized CPT code, authorized ICP-10 code, authorized provider NPI, authorized facility, and authorized date range into your tracking system. Any change to any of these fields before the service date triggers an auth update request.

2. Establish a standing process for locum tenens and covering provider situations: if a different provider may render the service, verify whether the auth is provider-specific or group-specific. Request a group-level auth when possible.

3. For surgical cases: have the surgical coordinator verify the authorized CPT code against the planned procedure at the time of surgical scheduling, not just at the time of auth request. Surgical plans change. Auth must track with those changes.

4. Implement a pre-service auth verification checklist: the day before any authorized service, verify that the auth number, CPT code, provider, facility, and date are all consistent with the planned service.

Type 3: Expired Authorization

CO-24	**Service Rendered After Authorization Expired**	**Frequency:** Moderate — especially common in surgical scheduling	**Appeal rate:** Low to Moderate: 25-45%. Prevention is far more effective than appeal.

An expired authorization denial is the most preventable of the three types because the expiration date is known at the time the authorization is issued. If the practice's tracking system includes auth expiration dates and generates alerts before they occur, this denial should essentially never happen.

The reality is that most practices track authorization numbers but not expiration dates. The auth gets filed, the appointment gets scheduled, and nobody checks whether the appointment date falls within the authorized window until the claim comes back denied.

FIX IT: What to do with this denial today

1. Check whether the payer will extend the authorization dates retroactively. Some payers allow a brief extension (5-10 business days) by phone when the expiration was due to scheduling factors outside the patient's control, such as a facility cancellation or a physician illness. Call the auth department, explain the circumstances, and request a date extension.

2. If retroactive extension is not available: appeal with documentation of the scheduling circumstances. Attach any records showing the appointment was rescheduled by the facility or provider rather than at the patient's request.

3. Request a new authorization for the service and resubmit the claim with the new auth number. Note that a new auth may require the payer to re-review medical necessity criteria, and approval is not guaranteed.

4. If all appeal paths fail: discuss with the patient. Depending on your contract and whether the patient was informed of the auth situation in advance, some cost recovery from the patient may be possible.

PREVENT IT: What to change so it stops happening

1. Track auth expiration dates in your practice management system alongside auth numbers. Every auth entered into the system should include: auth number, authorized service, authorized provider, authorized facility, authorized date range start, and authorized date range end.

2. Set automated alerts at 14 days and 7 days before auth expiration for any auth attached to a scheduled appointment. The alert triggers a check: is the appointment scheduled within the auth window? If not, renew the auth before the expiration date.

3. For services with long lead times (surgery, specialty procedures): request auth for a broader date range from the start when the payer allows it. Some payers will authorize a 60 or 90-day window rather than a specific date.

4. When a scheduled appointment is rescheduled to a date outside the current auth window: the rescheduling triggers an immediate auth renewal request. Build this into your scheduling workflow as a mandatory step.

5. Conduct a weekly auth expiration report: pull all open authorizations expiring within the next 30 days and match them against the appointment schedule. Any auth without a scheduled appointment within its window is either renewed or the appointment is confirmed.

The Auth Request That Gets Approved: What to Include

The quality of the authorization request determines the approval rate. A complete, well-documented request is processed faster and approved more often than a minimal submission that requires the payer to request additional information.

PRIOR AUTHORIZATION REQUEST — REQUIRED ELEMENTS

Patient information: Full name, date of birth, member ID, group number, and plan name exactly as they appear on the insurance card.

Ordering provider: Name, NPI (10-digit), specialty, and contact information. Some payers require the DEA number for certain medication authorizations.

Rendering provider (if different): For referrals and surgeries where the rendering provider differs from the ordering provider: include the rendering provider's name, NPI, and tax ID.

Facility: Name, NPI, address, and tax ID of the facility where the service will be performed. Required for procedures and surgeries — often omitted for office-based services.

Service requested: CPT code(s) with full description. For surgeries: include primary and all anticipated secondary procedure codes. An authorization that covers only the primary procedure will produce a mismatch denial on secondary codes.

Diagnosis: ICD-10-CM code(s) with description. Must be the most specific code available for the confirmed diagnosis. Unspecified codes increase denial risk.

Clinical documentation: Office notes supporting medical necessity, relevant lab results, imaging reports, prior treatment attempts, and any payer-specific clinical criteria documentation (e.g., step therapy requirements, conservative treatment failure records).

Requested date range: The anticipated service date and the range within which the service may occur. Request a range rather than a single date when the exact date is not yet confirmed.

The Auth Tracking Log: One Tool, Most Problems Solved

The single most effective tool for prior authorization management is a tracking log that is updated in real time and reviewed weekly. The following structure covers every field that matters. This can be maintained in a spreadsheet, in your practice management system, or in a dedicated auth tracking module.

Field	Purpose and What to Enter
Patient name + DOB	Identifies the patient. Use full name and date of birth to avoid confusion in practices with similar patient names.
Payer + plan name	Identifies the specific plan, not just the payer company. Auth requirements differ between a payer's HMO and PPO plans even when the payer name is the same.
CPT code(s) authorized	The exact procedure codes covered by this authorization. If multiple codes are covered, list all of them. Any code not listed is not authorized.
Auth number	The reference number issued by the payer upon approval. This goes on every claim for the authorized service.
Authorized provider NPI	The NPI of the provider for whom the auth was issued. A different rendering provider generates a Type 2 mismatch denial.
Authorized facility NPI	The NPI of the facility where the service is authorized to occur. Required for procedures and surgeries.
Auth start date	The first date on which the authorized service can be rendered. Services before this date are not covered by the auth.
Auth end date	The last date on which the authorized service can be rendered. Flag this date for renewal alerts at 14 and 7 days.
Date auth requested	The date your office submitted the auth request. Used to track payer turnaround time and escalate if approval is delayed.

Date auth received	The date you received the auth approval or denial. Used to confirm the auth is in hand before confirming the appointment.
Status	Current status: Pending / Approved / Denied / Expired / Renewed. Reviewed weekly — any pending auth beyond the payer's stated turnaround time triggers a follow-up call.
Notes	Free text for call records, follow-up actions, appeal status, and retro-auth outcomes.

WEEKLY AUTH REVIEW: Every week: (1) Pull all auths expiring within 30 days and match against the appointment schedule. Renew or confirm. (2) Pull all pending auths older than the payer's standard turnaround time (typically 3-5 business days for urgent, 14 business days for routine). Call the payer to escalate. (3) Pull all approved auths with no appointment scheduled. Confirm whether the service is still planned. The weekly review takes 30-45 minutes and prevents the majority of Type 2 and Type 3 auth denials.

An authorization is not a guarantee of payment. It is a statement that the service appears to meet coverage criteria based on the information submitted. The claim still has to be coded correctly, filed on time, and matched to the auth exactly.

CHAPTER 7 · PART 2: THE 12 DENIAL TYPES DECODED

Medical Necessity Denials

CO-50, CO-57 — the payer says it wasn't needed

When a payer denies a claim as not medically necessary, it is not making a clinical judgment about the quality of the physician's care. It is making an administrative determination that the documentation submitted with or attached to the claim does not satisfy the coverage criteria in its policy for that service. The distinction matters because it changes the response.

The physician may have made the correct clinical decision. The service may have been exactly what the patient needed. None of that is visible to the payer's adjudication system if the documentation does not say so in the right terms and connect the clinical findings to the coverage criteria in the right way. Medical necessity denials are documentation and communication failures as much as they are billing problems.

This chapter explains how payers define medical necessity, how to find and use the coverage policies that govern these denials, and how to write the appeal letter that wins.

What 'Medical Necessity' Actually Means to a Payer

The phrase 'medically necessary' sounds clinical. In the payer context it is contractual. Every payer defines medical necessity in its provider manual and applies that definition when adjudicating claims. While the exact wording varies, most definitions share the same core elements:

Element	What the Payer Is Looking For
Appropriate for the diagnosis	The service must be consistent with the established or working diagnosis. A service that would be appropriate for Diagnosis A but is billed with Diagnosis B fails this criterion regardless of clinical intent.
Consistent with accepted standards of care	The service must reflect what a reasonable physician would provide for the condition, based on current clinical evidence and professional society guidelines. Experimental or unproven treatments face higher scrutiny.
Not primarily for the convenience of the patient or provider	The service must be driven by clinical need, not scheduling convenience or patient preference. Inpatient admission that could have been handled outpatient is a common example.
The least costly alternative that is adequate	If a less expensive service would achieve the same clinical outcome, the more expensive service may be denied. Applies frequently to imaging (MRI vs X-ray), setting of care (inpatient vs outpatient), and medication selection.
Supported by documentation in the medical record	The documentation must affirmatively demonstrate each of the above elements. The payer does not assume clinical necessity — it must be stated and supported in the record.

> *The payer does not deny that the service happened. It denies that the documentation proves it needed to happen.*

CO-50 vs CO-57: Two Denial Codes, Same Problem

Code	Official Description	In Practice
CO-50	Non-covered service because it is not deemed a medical necessity by the payer	The payer reviewed the claim and determined the service does not meet medical necessity criteria based on the diagnosis submitted and/or the documentation available. The most common medical necessity denial code.
CO-57	Payment denied/reduced because the payer deems the information submitted does not support this level of service	Typically appears on E/M downcode denials — the payer has determined the documentation supports a lower level of service than was billed. The physician billed 99215 but the payer paid at 99213. The difference becomes a CO-57 adjustment.

> **CO-57 AND E/M DOWNCODING:** When CO-57 appears on an E/M claim, the payer has performed a medical record review and concluded the documentation does not support the level billed. This is different from a simple CO-50 denial — the payer has already seen the record and made a determination. The appeal must address the specific elements the payer found insufficient: medical decision making complexity, time documentation, or the history and examination elements that were present but not clearly documented.

LCD and NCD: The Coverage Policies That Govern These Denials

Every medical necessity denial is governed by a coverage policy. For Medicare, these are formalized as Local Coverage Determinations (LCDs) and National Coverage Determinations (NCDs). For commercial payers, they are called medical policies or coverage policies. Understanding and using these documents is the single most important skill in medical necessity appeal writing.

Policy Type	Who Issues It	How to Find and Use It
NCD (National Coverage Determination)	Centers for Medicare and Medicaid Services (CMS). Applies to all Medicare contractors nationwide.	Search cms.gov for 'NCD' plus the service name or CPT code. NCDs specify which diagnoses and clinical criteria must be present for Medicare to cover the service nationally.
LCD (Local Coverage Determination)	Medicare Administrative Contractors (MACs) — the regional contractors that process Medicare claims in your area. Each MAC may have different LCDs for the same service.	Go to cms.gov/medicare-coverage-database and search by your MAC jurisdiction and the CPT code. The LCD lists the ICD-10 codes considered covered indications and the documentation requirements. This is the most specific and most useful document for Medicare appeals.
Commercial medical policy	Each commercial payer develops its own medical policies. UnitedHealthcare, Aetna, BCBS, Cigna, Humana, and others each publish their policies on their provider portals.	Log into the payer's provider portal and search the medical policy library for the service name or CPT code. Match the clinical criteria in the policy against what is documented in the medical record. The gap between what the policy requires and what the record documents is exactly what the appeal letter must address.

Medicaid coverage policy	Each state's Medicaid program sets its own coverage criteria, often through coverage bulletins or provider manuals.	Access through your state Medicaid agency's provider portal or website. Medicaid policies often require specific prior treatment steps (step therapy) before the requested service is covered.

THE MOST COMMON APPEAL MISTAKE: Writing a medical necessity appeal without first reading the payer's coverage policy for the denied service. The appeal letter must address the specific criteria in the policy — not general clinical reasoning. A well-written letter that argues convincingly for clinical appropriateness but does not reference the payer's own policy criteria will frequently fail. The policy is the scorecard. The appeal letter answers each item on it.

CO-50: The Appeal Letter That Works

CO-50	**Not Medically Necessary**	**Frequency:** High — significant revenue exposure per claim	**Appeal rate:** Moderate to High: 55-70% with complete documentation and policy-matched letter

A successful CO-50 appeal does three things: it references the payer's own coverage policy, it connects the clinical documentation to each criterion in that policy, and it is brief enough to be read completely. Appeals that run to seven pages of clinical narrative are less effective than a focused three-paragraph letter attached to the right supporting documentation.

The Three-Paragraph Appeal Letter Structure

MEDICAL NECESSITY APPEAL LETTER — THREE-PARAGRAPH STRUCTURE

Paragraph 1 — Identify the claim and state the basis for appeal:

We are writing to appeal the denial of claim [claim number] for patient [name], date of service [date], for CPT code [code]. The claim was denied under CO-50 (not medically necessary). We respectfully disagree with this determination and are providing the following documentation in support of medical necessity under [Payer Name]'s coverage policy for [service name], Policy Number [X] or LCD [L-number].

Paragraph 2 — Connect the documentation to the policy criteria, point by point:

The patient presented with [diagnosis/ICD-10 code], which is identified as a covered indication under Section [X] of the referenced policy. The attached [office note / operative report / imaging report] dated [date] documents: [list the specific clinical findings that satisfy each coverage criterion in the policy, using the policy's own language where possible]. [If step therapy is required]: Prior conservative treatment was attempted as follows: [treatment, dates, outcome]. The patient failed to respond to [X] after [timeframe], as documented in the attached [record].

Paragraph 3 — State the request and the action needed:

Based on the documentation provided, this service meets all criteria established in [payer]'s medical necessity policy for [service]. We respectfully request that this claim be reconsidered and approved for payment of $[amount]. Please contact [name] at [phone] with any questions or to request additional documentation. If this appeal is denied, we request a written explanation identifying which specific clinical criteria were not met.

THE LAST SENTENCE IS IMPORTANT: Requesting a written explanation of which specific criteria were not met does two things: it holds the payer to a higher standard of specificity in the denial response, and it gives you the exact information you need to build a second-level appeal if the first is denied. Many payers will provide a more detailed explanation when formally requested in the appeal letter.

Documentation to Attach to the Appeal

- The relevant portions of the medical record: the office note(s) documenting the clinical findings that support medical necessity. Highlight or underline the specific language that addresses each coverage criterion. Reviewers read dozens of appeals per day — make it easy to find the relevant text.
- The payer's own coverage policy or LCD: attach a copy with the relevant criteria highlighted. This demonstrates that you have read the policy and are responding to its specific requirements.
- Supporting clinical literature: for services that are newer or less commonly performed, attaching a relevant clinical guideline from a professional society (AHA, ACC, AAOS, etc.) that supports the service strengthens the appeal.
- Prior treatment records (if step therapy was required): for services that require documentation of failed conservative treatment, attach the records showing what was tried, for how long, and the clinical outcome.
- Imaging or lab results: for diagnostic imaging denials, attach the reports that document the clinical findings justifying the study.

CO-57: E/M Downcode Appeals

CO-57	**Documentation Does Not Support Level Billed**	**Frequency:** Moderate — most common in high-volume E/M practices	**Appeal rate:** Moderate: 45-60% at first level; higher at peer review

When CO-57 appears on an E/M claim, the payer's clinical reviewer has determined that the medical record does not support the complexity level billed. The claim was paid at a lower level, and the difference was adjusted under CO-57. This is a post-payment determination, meaning payment was made at the lower level — you are appealing for the additional amount.

The 2021 E/M Documentation Standards

Since January 1, 2021, E/M level selection for office visits is based on either medical decision making (MDM) or total time. Understanding both methods is essential for CO-57 appeals, because the appeal must demonstrate that the documented level was appropriate under at least one of these two pathways.

MDM Level	Problems Addressed	Data Reviewed / Ordered	Risk of Complications
Straightforward	1 self-limited or minor problem	Minimal or none	Minimal risk — OTC medications, minor surgery
Low	2+ self-limited, or 1 stable chronic condition	Limited: review prior records or test results	Low risk — Rx drug management for established condition
Moderate	1 or more chronic conditions with exacerbation / new problem with additional workup	Moderate: independent interpretation of test, discussion with other provider	Moderate risk — new Rx, minor surgery with risk factors, hospitalization
High	Chronic conditions with severe exacerbation / threat to life or bodily function	Extensive: independent interpretation, discussion with external provider, review of prior external notes	High risk — drug therapy requiring intensive monitoring, decision re hospitalization or DNR

A CO-57 appeal for an E/M downcode should identify which MDM level was documented (or the total time documented if time-based billing was used), cite the specific clinical elements in the record that support that level, and explain how those elements meet the criteria for the billed code. If the payer downgraded from 99215 to 99213, the appeal must show that the encounter involved at least moderate MDM — two or more of the three MDM elements at the moderate level.

FIX IT: What to do with this denial today

1. Pull the denied claim and the payer's denial explanation. If CO-57, identify the specific level the payer paid at and the level that was billed.

2. For CO-50: locate the payer's coverage policy or LCD for the denied service. Read the covered indications and documentation requirements. Compare against the medical record.

3. For CO-57: review the E/M documentation using the 2021 MDM criteria table. Identify which MDM level the documentation supports. If it supports the billed level: build the appeal around the specific MDM elements present.

4. Write the appeal letter using the three-paragraph structure above. Attach the relevant medical record pages with the key clinical findings highlighted.

5. Submit within the payer's appeal deadline (typically 30-180 days from the denial date). If a first-level appeal is denied, request a second-level appeal (peer-to-peer review if available for CO-57).

6. For CO-57 specifically: request a peer-to-peer review with the payer's medical reviewer. Many payers allow the treating physician to speak directly with the reviewer. Peer-to-peer reviews have significantly higher overturn rates than written appeals alone.

PREVENT IT: What to change so it stops happening

1. Obtain the relevant LCD or commercial coverage policy for every service your practice performs regularly that carries medical necessity risk. Build a reference library organized by CPT code. For each service, document the covered ICD-10 codes and the required documentation elements.

2. Implement a pre-billing documentation check for high-risk services: before coding and submitting a claim for a service with known medical necessity risk (advanced imaging, injections, high-level E/M), verify that the medical record addresses each coverage criterion.

3. For E/M level selection: implement a documentation template or structured note that prompts the physician to address the MDM elements clearly. The most common CO-57 cause is not that the work was not done — it is that the work was not documented in a way that maps to the MDM criteria.

4. Train physicians on the specific documentation language that satisfies coverage criteria for your most commonly denied services. Clinical language that clearly supports the indication is more effective than comprehensive narrative that buries the key facts.

5. Track medical necessity denial rates by CPT code and by physician. A service or provider with a consistently elevated denial rate signals a documentation pattern that should be addressed before more claims go out.

Diagnosis Linking: The Fastest Fix for CO-50

The single most common and most fixable cause of CO-50 denials is a broken or absent link between the diagnosis code and the procedure code. The ICD-10 code submitted on the claim must be one that the payer's policy recognizes as a covered indication for the procedure. If it is not, the claim fails medical necessity even if the diagnosis is clinically correct.

This is a coding problem with a coding fix. The solution is not always a documentation fix or an appeal — sometimes it is a corrected claim with a more appropriate ICD-10 code.

Diagnosis Linking Scenario	What to Do

The ICD-10 submitted is correct but not on the LCD covered diagnosis list	Check whether a different ICD-10 code more accurately describes the documented condition AND appears on the covered diagnosis list. If the documentation supports the more specific code: submit a corrected claim. If the diagnosis genuinely does not appear on the LCD list: appeal with documentation arguing that the patient's condition is clinically equivalent to a covered indication.
The ICD-10 submitted is too non-specific (unspecified code used)	Look up the most specific ICD-10 code for the documented condition. If the medical record supports a more specific code: submit a corrected claim with the specific code. Many LCDs cover the specific code but not the unspecified version.
Multiple diagnoses present but only one submitted on the claim	Review the medical record for all active diagnoses relevant to the service. If a covered diagnosis exists in the record but was not submitted on the claim: submit a corrected claim with the additional diagnosis code in the correct position.
The primary diagnosis does not support the procedure but a secondary diagnosis does	ICD-10 code sequencing matters. The diagnosis most directly related to the service performed should appear first. If a secondary diagnosis supports the procedure better than the primary: resequence the diagnosis codes on a corrected claim.

CORRECTED CLAIM VS APPEAL: When the fix is a coding correction — a more specific ICD-10 code, a resequenced diagnosis list, or an additional code that was omitted — submit a corrected claim rather than an appeal. A corrected claim is processed faster, does not consume your appeal window, and does not require a letter. Reserve the appeal for situations where the documentation, not the coding, is the basis for the denial.

Step Therapy and Conservative Treatment Requirements

Many payer policies require documentation that conservative or less expensive treatments were attempted and failed before the requested service will be covered. This is called step therapy or fail-first protocol. It is particularly common for specialty drugs, advanced imaging, interventional pain procedures, and surgical interventions.

A CO-50 denial for a service subject to step therapy almost always means one of three things: the step therapy was not performed, the step therapy was performed but not documented, or the documentation of the step therapy was not included with the claim or auth request.

Step Therapy Situation	Correct Response
Step therapy was completed but not documented	Request the records from the treating provider who managed the prior treatment. Attach them to the appeal with a cover letter explaining the timeline of treatment attempts and outcomes.
Step therapy was completed and documented, but records were not submitted	Submit the appeal with the complete step therapy documentation. Reference the payer's policy requirement and demonstrate point-by-point compliance.
Step therapy was not completed because it was clinically contraindicated	Document the contraindication clearly in the appeal. Most payer policies include an exception for contraindicated step therapy. The documentation must explicitly state why the standard first-line treatment could not be used.
Step therapy was not completed because the physician was not aware of the requirement	This is a process gap, not an appeal basis. The appeal is likely to fail. Use this case to update your service-specific auth and documentation checklist so the step therapy requirement is captured before the next similar service.

> *The physician made the right call. The documentation has to prove it in the payer's language, not the physician's.*

CHAPTER 8 · PART 2: THE 12 DENIAL TYPES DECODED

Timely Filing Denials

CO-29 — the denial that is always 100% preventable

Every other denial category in this book involves some complexity. Maybe the coding was wrong. Maybe the documentation was insufficient. Maybe the payer applied the wrong coverage policy. There is usually something to investigate, something to argue, something to fix on the clinical or administrative side.

CO-29 is different. A timely filing denial means the claim was submitted after the payer's allowed window. There is no clinical argument to make. There is no documentation issue to address. The service was rendered, it was covered, and the practice did not submit the claim in time. The money is almost always gone.

The title of this chapter calls CO-29 always 100% preventable. That is not hyperbole. Unlike eligibility denials, which can occur when a payer retroactively terminates coverage, or medical necessity denials, which involve clinical judgment calls, a timely filing denial has one cause: a claim that was not submitted within the required timeframe. That is entirely within the billing team's control.

This chapter covers the filing windows by payer type, the narrow circumstances where an appeal can succeed, and the prevention system that eliminates this denial category permanently.

Filing Deadlines by Payer Type

CO-29	Timely Filing Limit Exceeded	**Frequency:** Low frequency in well-run practices; High cost when it occurs	**Appeal rate:** Very Low: 15-25% in narrow circumstances only

Every payer sets its own timely filing requirement. The deadline is measured from the date of service, not the date the claim was prepared or the date the patient was billed. The following table covers the standard windows — always verify the specific requirement in your payer contract, as commercial payer windows vary significantly.

Payer Type	Standard Filing Window	Notes and Exceptions
Medicare Part B (Physician / outpatient)	1 calendar year from the date of service	The Medicare timely filing window is one of the most generous in the industry. Claims for dates of service in 2024 must be submitted by December 31, 2025. No exceptions for late submission exist unless a very narrow set of administrative error exceptions apply (see Section 8.3).
Medicare Advantage (Part C plans)	Varies: typically 90 days to 1 year depending on the plan	Medicare Advantage plans are not bound by the same rules as traditional Medicare. Each plan sets its own window. Some are as short as 90 days. Always verify the specific MA plan's contract. Never assume MA follows traditional Medicare rules.

Medicaid	Varies significantly by state: 90 days to 1 year	Medicaid timely filing requirements are set at the state level. Some states require submission within 90 days of service. Others allow up to 12 months. Know your state's specific requirement and the rules for encounters involving third-party liability.
Commercial payers (major carriers)	90 days to 1 year; most commonly 90-180 days	UnitedHealthcare, Aetna, Cigna, BCBS, and Humana typically require submission within 90 to 180 days of service. The specific window is in the provider contract. When in doubt: assume 90 days and submit earlier.
TRICARE / CHAMPVA	1 year from the date of service for most claims	Similar to Medicare in generosity. Secondary claims (when TRICARE is secondary) have a 90-day window from the date of the primary payer's EOB.
Workers' Compensation	Varies by state: often 30-90 days, some states up to 1 year	Workers' compensation timely filing rules are set by state law, not payer contracts. Some states impose strict 30-day windows. Non-compliance can result in permanent forfeiture of the right to collect. Always confirm the state-specific deadline before treating a workers' comp patient.
Secondary payer (any payer type)	Typically 90 days from the primary payer's EOB date	When billing a secondary payer, the timely filing window usually begins when the primary EOB is received, not the date of service. Always include the primary EOB with the secondary claim. Confirm the secondary payer's specific rule.

PAYER CONTRACT IS THE AUTHORITY: The table above reflects standard industry windows. Your actual contractual obligation is in your provider agreement with each payer. When a payer's portal or the contract specifies a different window than what is listed here: the contract governs. Pull your contracts and document the timely filing window for every payer you bill. Update this reference whenever a contract renews.

What Resets the Clock

The timely filing window does not always start on the date of service. Several circumstances reset or extend the filing clock. Understanding these exceptions is the difference between a winnable appeal and a permanent write-off.

Circumstance	How It Affects the Filing Window
Coordination of benefits (COB) — secondary billing	When a patient has primary and secondary insurance, the secondary payer's timely filing window typically begins on the date the primary payer's EOB is received, not the date of service. Submit to the primary payer promptly so the secondary window does not begin with most of your secondary billing time already consumed.
Retroactive eligibility determination	When a patient's coverage is confirmed retroactively — for example, when a Medicaid application is approved weeks after the service date — the filing window for the now-covered claim may begin on the date eligibility was confirmed, not the date of service. Contact the payer to verify the applicable filing window in this situation.
Patient initially self-pay, later provides insurance	If a patient was treated as self-pay and subsequently provides insurance information, most payers allow submission within the standard filing window from the date the insurance information was received, not the date of service. Document when the insurance information was provided.

Coordination with workers' compensation or liability insurance	When a claim is pending resolution of a workers' compensation or liability claim, the group health payer's filing window may be extended until the liability decision is made. This varies significantly by state and by contract — confirm with the payer in writing before relying on this exception.
Corrected claim or adjustment	When a corrected claim is submitted to fix an error on a previously processed claim, most payers require the corrected claim within a defined window from the date of the original EOB (typically 90-180 days), not from the original date of service. Always verify the corrected claim deadline separately from the original filing deadline.
Administrative error by the payer	If the original claim was submitted within the timely filing window and was lost or misrouted by the payer or clearinghouse through no fault of the provider, the filing clock may be stopped or extended. This is a narrow exception that requires proof of original timely submission.

When a Timely Filing Appeal Can Win

The appeal success rate for CO-29 denials is low because the majority of them reflect genuine late submission. However, a small but meaningful category of timely filing denials is appealable — and winning these appeals requires one thing above all else: proof of original timely submission.

Winnable Timely Filing Appeal Scenarios

Scenario	What You Need to Win

Claim was submitted on time but the payer has no record of receiving it	Clearinghouse acknowledgment report showing the claim was accepted and forwarded to the payer within the filing window. This is the strongest evidence available. If the clearinghouse confirms timely forwarding and the payer lost the claim, the denial is the payer's administrative error — appealable.
Claim was submitted on time but was rejected by the clearinghouse for a technical error	The original submission date on the clearinghouse report plus a record of the rejection notice and the correction and resubmission dates. If the technical error was minor and the resubmission occurred promptly, some payers will honor the original submission date for timely filing purposes.
Retroactive eligibility change extended the filing window	Documentation of when eligibility was retroactively confirmed, and the payer's written policy or contract language stating that the filing window begins at eligibility confirmation. Include both with the appeal.
COB secondary claim filed within the window from the primary EOB date	The primary EOB date plus your submission date, showing the secondary claim was filed within the contractual window from that date. Include a copy of the primary EOB.
State or federal disaster or public health emergency extended the deadline	CMS and some commercial payers issue blanket timely filing waivers during declared emergencies. If the date of service falls within a waiver period: cite the specific waiver, its effective dates, and your submission date. Attach the waiver documentation.

THE ONE DOCUMENT THAT WINS TIMELY FILING APPEALS: The clearinghouse acknowledgment report — specifically, the 277CA (Claims Acknowledgment) transaction or its equivalent — is proof that your claim was received by the clearinghouse and forwarded to the payer within the filing window. Save every clearinghouse acknowledgment for every claim submitted. This is the document that converts an unwinnable timely filing denial into a winnable administrative error appeal. If your clearinghouse does not provide downloadable acknowledgment reports, switch to one that does or enable that feature in your current system.

The Timely Filing Appeal Letter

A timely filing appeal is one of the shortest appeal letters you will write because the argument is narrow: we submitted on time, and here is the proof. The letter should be direct and the documentation should be unambiguous.

TIMELY FILING APPEAL LETTER — TEMPLATE

We are writing to appeal the denial of claim [claim number] for patient [name], date of service [date], CPT code [code], denied under CO-29 (timely filing limit exceeded).

This claim was submitted to [payer name] within the required filing window. Attached is the clearinghouse acknowledgment report confirming that the claim was transmitted on [submission date], which is within the [X]-day filing requirement for dates of service on [DOS]. The claim was [accepted by the clearinghouse and forwarded to your system / returned to us for correction on (date), corrected and resubmitted on (date)].

[If applicable: This claim was initially processed as self-pay because the patient did not provide insurance information at the time of service. Insurance information was received on [date], and the claim was submitted within [X] days of that date, consistent with your policy for late insurance disclosure.]

We respectfully request that this denial be reversed and the claim be reprocessed for payment. Please contact [name] at [phone] if additional documentation is required.

The Prevention System: Why This Denial Should Never Appear

A practice that receives CO-29 denials has a workflow problem, not a billing knowledge problem. The knowledge that claims must be submitted within a defined window is universal. The failure is in the tracking system that allows claims to age past that window without triggering action.

The following prevention system has three components. All three are necessary. Any one of them alone is insufficient.

Component 1: The Claim Age Report

Every practice management system generates a claim age report — a list of all submitted claims organized by how many days have passed since the date of service. If yours does not, it is the most important report to configure. Run it weekly without exception.

Age Bucket	Claim Status	Required Action
0-30 days	Submitted, awaiting adjudication	Monitor for clearinghouse acknowledgment. No action needed unless no acknowledgment received.
31-60 days	Should be adjudicated or pending	Check claim status in payer portal. If still pending: note and monitor. If no record found at payer: investigate submission and consider resubmission.
61-90 days	Approaching the danger zone for 90-day payers	For any payer with a 90-day window: escalate immediately. Contact the payer, confirm receipt of the claim, and document the call. If the claim is not found: resubmit immediately with proof of original submission.

91-120 days	Timely filing risk zone for most commercial payers	For commercial payers: determine whether the claim is still within the filing window. If not: assess whether an appeal is viable. If within window: resubmit now with no further delay.
121-180 days	High risk. Medicare still within window; many commercial payers are not.	For Medicare: still submittable. For commercial payers with 90-180 day windows: final submission opportunity. Act immediately.
181-365 days	Most commercial payers closed. Medicare still open (if within 1 year of DOS).	For Medicare: submit immediately if within the calendar year window. For commercial payers: assess appeal viability. Most commercial claims past 180 days have limited recovery options.

Component 2: The Weekly Audit Workflow

The claim age report is the data. The weekly audit is the process that acts on it. Assign a specific person or team to run the age report every week and take action on every claim in the 61-day-and-older buckets before the week ends. This is not optional and it is not something that can be done monthly. Claims age every day. The audit must match the pace.

WEEKLY TIMELY FILING AUDIT — FOUR STEPS

Step 1: Run the claim age report filtered to show all unpaid claims 60 days or older. Sort by payer.

Step 2: For each payer in the report: identify the timely filing deadline. Flag any claim approaching within 30 days of that deadline as urgent.

Step 3: For each flagged claim: check the payer portal for current claim status. If pending: document and monitor. If not found: initiate resubmission immediately with clearinghouse proof of original submission.

Step 4: Document the audit in your billing log: date run, number of claims reviewed, number escalated, actions taken. This log is your evidence of due diligence if a timely filing appeal is ever needed.

Component 3: The Submission Confirmation Habit

Every claim submitted must generate a confirmation that it was received. This is not an optional step. It is the proof that protects your appeal rights if the payer later claims the claim was not received on time.

- For electronic submissions: save or archive the clearinghouse 277CA acknowledgment for every claim batch. Most practice management systems store these automatically — confirm yours does and that the records are accessible for at least two years.
- For paper submissions: submit by certified mail with return receipt. The USPS tracking confirmation is your proof of timely submission. This applies to any payer that still requires paper claims.
- For payer portal submissions: print or save a PDF of the submission confirmation page before navigating away. Portal submission records are not always accessible retroactively, and the confirmation page is the only proof you submitted if the claim later disappears from the payer's system.
- Archive all submission confirmations for at least two years from the date of service. Timely filing appeals can be filed months after the denial, and you need the original submission proof to be readily accessible when that happens.

FIX IT: What to do with this denial today

1. Verify whether an appeal is viable: gather your proof of original submission date (clearinghouse acknowledgment, certified mail tracking, portal confirmation page) and compare it to the payer's stated filing window.

2. If you have proof of timely submission: file the appeal immediately using the template above. Attach the submission proof as the primary exhibit. Keep the letter short — one page maximum. The documentation does the arguing.

3. If the submission was not timely and no clock-reset exception applies: assess write-off. Do not spend significant staff time appealing a genuinely late claim with no viable exception. The ROI on that effort is extremely low.

4. If a COB, retroactive eligibility, or late insurance disclosure exception may apply: document the circumstances in the appeal letter and include supporting records for the exception.

5. Document the outcome and the root cause in your denial log. A CO-29 denial is always a process failure. Knowing which part of the process failed prevents the same failure on the next claim.

PREVENT IT: What to change so it stops happening

1. Run the claim age report every week. Every week. No exceptions. This single habit, consistently executed, eliminates timely filing denials in most practices within 60-90 days of implementation.

2. Build a payer-specific filing deadline reference. For every payer you bill: document the timely filing window in your billing reference guide. Include Medicare (1 year), Medicare Advantage (plan-specific), Medicaid (state-specific), and each commercial contract. Review and update annually when contracts renew.

3. Save every clearinghouse acknowledgment automatically. Configure your practice management system or clearinghouse to archive 277CA acknowledgments and make them searchable by patient, date of service, and claim number.

4. Set filing deadline alerts in your practice management system for claims approaching the 60-day mark. The alert triggers a status check — not a resubmission, a check. Only resubmit if the claim is not found in the payer's system.

5. Assign timely filing accountability. One person or team owns the age report review. When everyone is responsible for timely filing, no one is. Assign it, schedule it, and review the outcomes monthly.

The ROI Calculation: When to Write Off vs When to Fight

Not every timely filing denial is worth the staff time required to investigate and appeal it. The following framework helps you make that decision quickly.

Claim Amount	Appeal Viability	Recommended Action
Any amount	High (proof of timely submission exists)	File the appeal. The documentation does most of the work. Estimated staff time: 30-60 minutes. Recovery rate: 70-80%.
Over $500	Moderate (COB, retro-eligibility, or disaster waiver exception may apply)	Investigate the exception, build the appeal if viable. Estimated staff time: 1-2 hours. Recovery rate: 25-45%.
Under $200	Low (no proof of timely submission, genuine late filing)	Write off. The staff time to investigate and appeal exceeds the likely recovery on a low-dollar claim with weak appeal grounds.
Over $500	Low (no proof of timely submission, genuine late filing)	Evaluate case-by-case. Consider a brief good-faith appeal letter referencing any mitigating circumstances. Outcome is unlikely but the dollar amount may justify the attempt.
Any amount	None (filing window missed by more than 30 days with no exceptions)	Write off immediately. Document the root cause. Use the failure to reinforce the prevention system.

> *A timely filing denial is not a billing problem. It is a tracking problem. Fix the tracking and the denial disappears.*

CHAPTER 9 · PART 2: THE 12 DENIAL TYPES DECODED

Modifier and Coding Denials

CO-4, CO-11, CO-22 — the code was wrong

Coding denials are the most controllable denial category in medical billing. Unlike eligibility denials, which depend on what the insurance company does, or medical necessity denials, which depend on what the physician documents, coding denials originate entirely within the billing and coding process. The wrong code was assigned, the wrong modifier was applied, or the claim was submitted to the wrong payer. All of these are fixable at the point of coding — before the claim goes out.

The three denial codes in this chapter — CO-4, CO-11, and CO-22 — collectively cover the most common coding-related reasons a claim is rejected or paid incorrectly. Each has a distinct meaning, a distinct cause, and a distinct fix. Understanding the difference between them is the first step toward a coding process that catches these problems before the payer does.

The Three Denial Codes: What Each One Actually Means

Code	Official Description	What Is Actually Wrong

CO-4	The procedure code is inconsistent with the modifier	A modifier was appended to a CPT code in a combination the payer does not accept. The modifier may not apply to this code, or the modifier requires documentation that was not present, or the wrong modifier was used for the clinical circumstance.
CO-11	The diagnosis is inconsistent with the procedure	The ICD-10 code submitted does not clinically or logically support the CPT code billed. The payer's editing system found the combination implausible or inconsistent with coverage criteria.
CO-22	This care may be covered by another payer	The claim was submitted to the wrong payer, or coordination of benefits applies and this payer believes another insurance should be primary. The claim cannot be adjudicated until the COB question is resolved.

CO-4: Procedure Code Inconsistent With Modifier

CO-4	**Procedure / Modifier Inconsistency**	**Frequency:** Very High — #1 or #2 denial in most practices	**Appeal rate:** Moderate: 50-65% with corrected claim or modifier documentation

CO-4 covering modifier inconsistency is distinct from CO-4 covering diagnosis-procedure inconsistency (which was addressed in Chapter 4). Here, the problem is specifically the modifier-to-code pairing. The payer's system encountered a combination it does not recognize as valid, or a modifier that requires clinical circumstances that were not documented.

The Most Common CO-4 Modifier Errors

Modifier	Error Pattern	Correct Approach
`-25 on procedure code`	Modifier -25 was appended to a procedure code rather than an E/M code. -25 applies only to E/M codes (99202-99499).	Remove -25 from the procedure code. If a separate E/M service was provided on the same day as the procedure, append -25 to the E/M code, not the procedure code.
`-51 exempt code + -51`	Modifier -51 (multiple procedures) was appended to a code that is exempt from -51 under the CPT add-on code or -51 exempt designation. Common with add-on codes like 99354 or 99355.	Remove -51 from exempt codes. Add-on codes are inherently priced as additional services and do not require -51. Check the CPT manual's -51 exempt list before appending.
`-59 without documentation basis`	Modifier -59 was used to separate two codes that are legitimately bundled under NCCI, but the clinical circumstances that justify separate billing (different anatomic site, different session) are not documented in the record.	If the services were genuinely performed separately: add documentation to the record and resubmit. If the services were not separately performed: the bundling is correct and -59 is not appropriate.
`-26 or -TC on global code`	The professional (-26) or technical component (-TC) modifier was appended to a code that does not have a professional/technical component split. Not all CPT codes can be split.	Verify whether the CPT code has a professional and technical component by checking the Medicare Physician Fee Schedule. If no split exists: remove the modifier and bill the global code.

`-LT/-RT on non-bilateral code`	Left (-LT) or right (-RT) modifiers were appended to a CPT code that is not a bilateral procedure code and does not accept these modifiers.	Verify whether the CPT code accepts -LT/-RT modifiers in the Medicare fee schedule or payer's policy. If not accepted: remove the modifier. For truly bilateral procedures: use modifier -50 instead.
`-GT or -95 (telehealth) on non-covered service`	A telehealth modifier was appended to a CPT code that the payer does not cover via telehealth for this patient's plan type or geographic location.	Verify payer-specific telehealth coverage before billing. Not all services are covered via telehealth and coverage varies by payer, plan type, and state. Remove the modifier if telehealth is not covered for this service.

The Global Surgical Package and Modifier Denials

The most common source of CO-4 modifier denials in surgical practices is the global surgical package combined with incorrect or missing modifiers. When a service is billed within the global period of a prior procedure without the correct modifier, the payer bundles it into the global package and denies the separate billing under CO-4 or CO-97.

Situation	Required Modifier	Documentation Required
E/M visit during global period for unrelated condition	`-24 on the E/M code`	The note must clearly document that the visit was for a condition unrelated to the original surgery. The chief complaint, diagnosis, and plan must be for a separate problem.

Staged or related procedure during global period	`-58 on the second procedure`	Documentation must show the second procedure was either planned prospectively at the time of the original surgery, is more extensive than the original, or is for therapy following the original diagnostic service.
Unrelated procedure during global period	`-79 on the second procedure`	Documentation must establish the second procedure was for a condition unrelated to the original surgery. Separate diagnosis, separate clinical indication.
Return to OR for complication (same surgeon)	`No additional modifier required — bill the return procedure code; payer may request records`	Document the complication clearly. The return to OR for a complication of the original procedure is generally included in the global package and not separately billable unless the complication is unrelated.

FIX IT: What to do with this denial today

1. Identify the specific modifier causing the CO-4. The remark code on the EOB often specifies which modifier was rejected. If not: call the payer and ask which modifier-code combination was flagged.

2. Determine whether the modifier was wrong for this code (remove it and resubmit without), or whether the modifier was right but the documentation was insufficient (add documentation and resubmit with the modifier).

3. For global period modifier denials: pull the original procedure date and calculate the global period (0, 10, or 90 days). Determine which modifier applies to the new service and whether the documentation supports it.

4. Submit a corrected claim with the modifier correction. Include a brief cover note if the modifier was removed or changed to help the payer process the correction without flagging a duplicate.

PREVENT IT: What to change so it stops happening

1. Build a modifier decision tree for your top 20 CPT codes. For each code: which modifiers are accepted, which are excluded, and what documentation is required for each accepted modifier. Post this at every coder's workstation.
2. Enable NCCI edit checking and payer-specific modifier validation in your clearinghouse or practice management system before claims are submitted.
3. For surgical practices: maintain a global period tracker for every procedure performed. Flag any new billing for the same patient within the global period and confirm the correct modifier before submission.
4. Conduct quarterly modifier audits: pull 10-15 claims per coder that included modifiers and verify the modifier was appropriate for the code and the documentation supports it.

CO-11: Diagnosis Inconsistent With Procedure

CO-11	**Diagnosis Does Not Support Procedure**	**Frequency:** High — among the most common denial codes	**Appeal rate:** Moderate to High: 60-70% with corrected diagnosis or documentation appeal

CO-11 is the diagnosis-procedure linking denial. The ICD-10 code submitted does not make clinical sense in combination with the CPT code billed — at least not according to the payer's automated editing logic. This is distinct from a medical necessity denial (CO-50), which involves a policy judgment about whether the service was needed. CO-11 is an internal consistency check: does the diagnosis explain why the procedure was performed?

Why CO-11 Happens: Four Patterns

Pattern	Example and Fix

Symptom code submitted when a definitive diagnosis is available	Symptom code R10.9 (unspecified abdominal pain) submitted with CPT 44950 (appendectomy). Once the appendectomy is performed, the diagnosis is K37 (unspecified appendicitis) — not the presenting symptom. Fix: use the confirmed diagnosis established by the end of the encounter, not the presenting symptom.
Wrong body system or site in the diagnosis	CPT 27447 (total knee arthroplasty, left) billed with ICD-10 M17.11 (primary osteoarthritis, right knee). The laterality of the diagnosis does not match the laterality of the procedure. Fix: verify the diagnosis code matches the operative side documented in the chart.
Diagnosis does not clinically indicate the procedure performed	CPT 71046 (chest X-ray, 2 views) billed with ICD-10 J00 (common cold). A payer's editing system may flag this as inconsistent because chest X-rays are not a standard diagnostic tool for a common cold. Fix: use the diagnosis that specifically prompted the imaging — e.g., R05.9 (cough) or J18.9 (pneumonia, unspecified) if pneumonia was suspected.
Outdated or deleted diagnosis code	An ICD-10 code that was valid in a prior year was used for a current date of service. Deleted codes produce CO-11 or technical rejections. Fix: look up the current-year replacement code and resubmit. Build an October 1 code update review into your annual workflow.

Sequencing: When the Right Code Is in the Wrong Position

ICD-10 diagnosis codes are submitted in a specific sequence on a claim. The primary diagnosis — the condition most responsible for the service — goes first. Additional diagnoses follow. When the code that supports the procedure is in a secondary position and the primary diagnosis does not logically relate to the procedure, CO-11 can result even when the correct code is present on the claim.

- The principal diagnosis should be the condition most directly linked to the service billed. If a patient is treated for both hypertension and a broken wrist in the same encounter, and the encounter was primarily for the wrist, the fracture code should be primary.

- Check the sequence before submission on any claim where multiple diagnoses are present. The payer's editing system evaluates the primary diagnosis against the primary procedure first.
- For claims denied with CO-11 where the correct diagnosis is present but sequenced incorrectly: submit a corrected claim with the diagnosis codes resequenced. This is one of the fastest fixes in billing.

FIX IT: What to do with this denial today

1. Pull the denied claim and identify both the diagnosis code and the procedure code that triggered CO-11.

2. Determine which of the four patterns applies: symptom vs definitive diagnosis, laterality mismatch, clinical inconsistency, or deleted code.

3. For symptom vs definitive diagnosis and laterality mismatches: submit a corrected claim with the corrected ICD-10 code. No appeal letter needed.

4. For clinical inconsistency denials where the documentation supports a different diagnosis: review the medical record, identify the more appropriate ICD-10 code, and submit a corrected claim.

5. For clinical inconsistency denials where the submitted diagnosis was correct and the payer's editing logic is wrong: appeal with a brief letter explaining the clinical relationship between the diagnosis and the procedure, citing any relevant LCD or coverage policy that lists the submitted ICD-10 as a covered indication.

6. For deleted code denials: look up the current ICD-10 replacement code and resubmit immediately.

PREVENT IT: What to change so it stops happening

1. Implement a diagnosis-procedure crosscheck at the point of coding: for every claim with a procedure code, verify that the primary diagnosis makes clinical sense as the reason for the procedure before submitting.

2. Maintain an updated ICD-10 coding reference for your top 25 most-billed procedures. For each procedure: list the accepted and commonly denied diagnosis pairings. Update annually on October 1.

3. Train coders on the distinction between symptom codes and definitive diagnosis codes. The general rule: use the most definitive diagnosis available at the end of the encounter. Symptom codes are appropriate only when no definitive diagnosis has been established.

4. Add laterality verification to your coding checklist for all orthopedic, ophthalmologic, ENT, and other bilateral-structure procedures. The diagnosis side must match the procedure side.

CO-22: Submitted to Wrong Payer / COB Applies

CO-22	**Coordination of Benefits — Another Payer May Be Primary**	**Frequency:** Moderate — common when COB is not verified at registration	**Appeal rate:** High: 75-85% once correct payer sequence is established

CO-22 tells you the claim landed in the wrong place. Either it was sent to a payer that is not responsible for it, or it was sent to a secondary payer without the primary payer's EOB attached, or the payer believes another insurer should be primary based on coordination of benefits rules. The fix is almost always straightforward once you identify the correct payer sequence.

Coordination of Benefits: The Rules That Determine Payer Order

When a patient has more than one insurance plan, coordination of benefits (COB) rules determine which plan pays first (primary) and which pays second (secondary). These rules are standardized across most payers through the NAIC Model COB Regulation, though individual payer contracts may modify them slightly.

COB Rule	How It Determines Primary Payer

Birthday rule (most common for dependent children)	When a child is covered by both parents' plans, the plan of the parent whose birthday (month and day, not year) falls earliest in the calendar year is primary. Example: Parent A's birthday is March 15. Parent B's birthday is August 3. Parent A's plan is primary for the child.
Employment status rule	Coverage through active employment is primary over coverage obtained through COBRA or retirement. If a patient has both an active employer plan and a COBRA plan, the active employer plan is primary.
Medicare as secondary payer (MSP)	Medicare is secondary when the patient has employer group health coverage through an employer with 20 or more employees (for patients under 65 on Medicare due to disability: 100 or more employees). Billing Medicare primary in these situations is a compliance violation.
No-fault / liability insurance	When treatment is related to an auto accident or liability claim, the no-fault or liability carrier is primary before any health insurance. Billing health insurance primary for accident-related care without resolving the liability question first generates CO-22.
Workers' compensation	Workers' compensation is always primary for work-related injuries. Health insurance cannot be billed primary for workers' comp claims. CO-22 appears when a health claim is submitted for a work-related injury without a workers' comp determination.

Medicare Secondary Payer: The Compliance Risk

MSP is worth special attention because billing Medicare primary when another payer should be primary is not just a denial issue — it is a compliance issue with potential repayment obligations and, in egregious cases, False Claims Act exposure. Always verify MSP status for Medicare patients who appear to have other insurance.

- The MSP questionnaire is required for all Medicare patients. If the patient has employer group health coverage through a current employer with 20 or more employees: that plan is primary, Medicare is secondary.
- Medicare's MSP Coordination of Benefits Contractor (COBC) can be contacted to verify a patient's MSP status and update the record if the wrong primary payer is on file.
- If Medicare was billed primary in error and paid: refund the Medicare payment and resubmit to the correct primary payer before billing Medicare as secondary.

FIX IT: What to do with this denial today

1. Identify whether the denial is a wrong-payer submission or a COB sequence issue. Call the payer that denied and ask: 'Which payer do you believe should be primary for this patient on this date?' Document the response.

2. For wrong-payer submissions: resubmit the claim to the correct primary payer immediately. The timely filing clock has been running since the date of service — do not delay.

3. For COB secondary denials where the primary EOB was not attached: resubmit to the secondary payer with the primary payer's EOB attached. Most secondary payers require the EOB as part of the claim submission.

4. For Medicare MSP situations where Medicare was billed primary in error: contact Medicare to report the error, refund the Medicare payment if one was made, submit to the correct primary payer, and then bill Medicare as secondary with the primary EOB.

5. For no-fault or workers' comp situations: determine whether a liability or workers' comp claim has been opened. If yes: submit to that carrier. If the patient denies a work or accident connection and health insurance was legitimately primary: document that determination in the chart.

PREVENT IT: What to change so it stops happening

1. Collect COB information at every registration and re-verify it annually. The COB question is: 'Do you have any other health insurance coverage, including coverage through a spouse, parent, employer, automobile insurance, or workers' compensation?'

2. For patients with Medicare: complete the MSP questionnaire at registration and update it whenever the patient's employment status changes.
3. Build a COB verification step into your eligibility verification process. Most real-time eligibility (270/271) responses include information about other payer coverage. Review this field for every patient.
4. For new patients with multiple insurances: determine the correct COB sequence before the first claim is submitted, not after the first denial.
5. Train front desk staff on the birthday rule and common COB scenarios for dependent children. This is the highest-frequency COB error in pediatric and family medicine practices.

The 10-Claim Monthly Coding Audit

Coding denials are best addressed at the source: the coding process itself. A monthly audit of a small sample of coded claims catches systematic errors before they become denial patterns. The audit does not need to be large to be effective – ten randomly selected claims per coder per month, reviewed against the medical record and the payer's coverage policies, identifies most recurring coding problems within two or three audit cycles.

THE 10-CLAIM MONTHLY CODING AUDIT

Step 1: Select the sample.

Pull 10 claims per coder from the prior month. Include a mix of claim types: at least two E/M-plus-procedure claims, two surgical claims, two multi-diagnosis claims, and four general office visit claims. Random selection is more revealing than cherry-picking.

Step 2: For each claim, verify five elements.

(1) Primary diagnosis is the condition most responsible for the service, and it logically supports the primary procedure. (2) All modifiers applied are appropriate for the specific CPT code used. (3) Diagnosis codes are current-year codes, not deleted or revised codes. (4) Laterality of diagnosis matches laterality of procedure where applicable. (5) No code pair on the claim is subject to an NCCI bundling edit that was not properly addressed with a modifier.

Step 3: Document findings.

Record each error found: the claim, the error type, and whether it resulted in a denial. Track error rates by coder and by error type over time. A coder with a high rate of modifier errors needs modifier training. A practice with a high rate of CO-11 denials on a specific procedure needs a diagnosis reference tool for that code.

Step 4: Feed findings back.

Share audit results with each coder in a brief monthly review. Frame errors as learning opportunities, not disciplinary issues. A coder who understands the pattern of their errors corrects faster than one who only receives a list of denied claims.

AUDIT SCOPE EXPANDER: Once your baseline coding audit is running smoothly, expand it to include high-dollar claims (over $1,000 billed) and claims for services with historically elevated denial rates. These two categories have the highest ROI for audit time: high-dollar claims because the per-error recovery is significant, and high-denial-rate services because systematic errors there affect every claim for that service.

> *A coding denial is the payer telling you what your coding process missed. The audit is how you hear that message before the claim goes out.*

CHAPTER 10 · PART 2: THE 12 DENIAL TYPES DECODED

Demographic and Data Entry Denials

CO-16, CO-M76 — the dumbest denials and how to stop them

The chapter title calls these the dumbest denials. That is not an insult — it is an acknowledgment that demographic and data entry denials are the most frustrating category in medical billing precisely because they have nothing to do with clinical care, coding expertise, or coverage policy. A patient's name was spelled wrong. A date of birth had two digits transposed. An NPI was missing from the referring provider field. The claim comes back denied, and somewhere between $50 and $5,000 of legitimate revenue is delayed or lost because of a clerical error that took three seconds to make and five minutes to fix.

What makes these denials worth a full chapter is the pattern. Every practice that tracks its denial data finds that demographic and data entry errors account for 15 to 20 percent of all denials, and that the same errors recur on the same types of claims from the same staff members. These are not random mistakes. They are systematic gaps in the registration and data entry process, and they respond well to systematic solutions.

CO-16 and CO-M76: What Each One Means

CO-16	Missing / Incorrect / Insufficient Information	**Frequency:** High — 15-20% of all denials in most practices	**Appeal rate:** Very High: 85-95% once the correct information is submitted

CO-16 is the most generic of all denial codes. It tells you something is missing, incorrect, or insufficient on the claim, but it does not specify what. The remark code attached to the CO-16 is where the actual information lives. Never respond to a CO-16 without first reading the remark code.

Code	What It Covers	Most Actionable With
CO-16	Claim/service lacks information or has submission/billing error(s). A catch-all for missing, incorrect, or insufficient data on the claim form itself.	Remark codes N115 (NPI required), N382 (invalid patient identifier), MA130 (additional information needed), N56 (procedure code not on file). Always read the remark code first.
CO-M76	Missing/incomplete/invalid diagnosis or procedure code(s). Specifically flags a problem with a code field rather than a demographic or administrative field.	Often appears alongside CO-16. The remark code specifies whether the diagnosis code, procedure code, or both are the issue. Treat as a corrected claim situation once the specific field is identified.

The Seven Most Common Data Entry Errors

The following seven errors produce the majority of CO-16 denials in outpatient physician billing. Each is presented with its most common cause, the remark code it typically generates, and the fix. Recognizing the pattern allows you to go directly to the correction without spending time investigating what went wrong.

Error Type	Typical Remark Code	Most Common Cause	Fix
Patient name mismatch	N382, CO-16	Name on the claim does not exactly match the name on file with the payer. Common causes: nickname vs legal name (Bob vs Robert), hyphenated surname entered without hyphen, suffix omitted (Jr., Sr.), maiden name on card vs married name in system.	Pull the physical insurance card or payer portal member record. Enter the name exactly as it appears — character for character including hyphens, spaces, and suffixes. Resubmit corrected claim.
Date of birth error	N382, CO-16	Single digit transposed (01/15 becomes 01/51), month and day swapped (03/12 becomes 12/03), or wrong year entered. Often occurs when staff reads a handwritten intake form incorrectly.	Verify DOB directly from the insurance card or a government-issued photo ID. Compare to the payer's member record via the eligibility portal. Correct and resubmit.

Member ID / subscriber ID error	N382, CO-16	ID copied incorrectly from the insurance card, leading zero dropped, letter confused with number (0 vs O, 1 vs I), or old ID entered from a prior plan year.	Scan the physical insurance card front and back. Verify the current member ID via real-time eligibility check. Never enter a member ID from verbal patient report without confirming against the card.
NPI missing or incorrect	N115, CO-16	Rendering provider NPI not populated, billing NPI used where rendering NPI is required, or individual NPI used where group NPI is required (or vice versa).	Identify which NPI is required: billing (group) NPI vs rendering (individual) NPI. Verify the correct NPI for each provider in the NPPES registry (nppes.cms.hhs.gov). Correct the specific NPI field and resubmit.
Referring provider identifier missing	MA130, CO-16	Referring provider NPI was not populated on the claim. Required for specialist and laboratory claims under Medicare and many commercial plans that require a PCP referral.	Obtain the referring provider's NPI from your records or from the NPPES registry. Add to the referring provider field and resubmit. For ongoing referral relationships: store the referring provider NPI in your system for automatic population.

Place of service code incorrect	CO-16, CO-4	Place of service (POS) code on the claim does not match where the service was actually rendered. Common: office (11) used when service was rendered at a patient's home (12), telehealth (02 or 10) not updated from the default office code, or outpatient hospital (22) vs office (11) mix-up.	Verify the actual location of service from the appointment record. Select the correct CMS place of service code for that location. For telehealth: POS 02 (telehealth, patient not at home) or POS 10 (telehealth, patient at home) depending on the patient's location during the visit.
Taxonomy code error	CO-16, N115	Billing provider taxonomy code does not match the specialty on file with the payer, or the taxonomy code does not match the type of service billed. Taxonomy codes identify provider specialty and type.	Verify the correct taxonomy code for the billing provider's specialty at nucc.org. Confirm the taxonomy code on file with each payer matches. Correct and resubmit. For new providers: establish the correct taxonomy code before the first claim is submitted.

The 45-Second Double-Check Workflow

The most effective prevention tool for demographic denials is a structured double-check at two points in the patient encounter: at check-in and at claim submission. The check-in verification catches errors before the service is rendered. The submission check catches errors before the claim goes to the payer. Together they eliminate most CO-16 denials without adding significant staff time.

THE 45-SECOND CHECK-IN VERIFICATION

Every patient, every visit — no exceptions for established patients.

1. Ask: 'Has your name, date of birth, or address changed since your last visit?' Do not assume the answer is no.

2. Ask: 'Do you have your insurance card with you today?' Scan or photograph both sides of the card even if the patient reports no changes. Cards are updated annually. Card images from a year ago may be wrong.

3. Compare the card to what is in the system: member ID character-by-character, group number, plan name, and patient name spelling. Correct any discrepancy before the patient leaves the front desk.

4. Run a real-time eligibility check. Confirm the member ID in the system returns a valid match in the payer's eligibility database. A successful 271 response is the final confirmation that the demographic data is correct.

THE PRE-SUBMISSION CLAIM REVIEW

Before any claim batch is transmitted to the clearinghouse:

1. Verify that the rendering provider NPI field is populated for every claim in the batch. Missing NPI is the most common field-level error on electronically submitted claims.

2. Verify the place of service code matches the actual service location. For telehealth claims: confirm the telehealth POS code (02 or 10) is in place, not the default office POS (11).

3. For specialist claims requiring a referring provider: verify the referring provider NPI is populated in the correct field.

4. Run the batch through your clearinghouse's claim scrubbing tool before transmitting. Most clearinghouses flag missing or invalid NPI, invalid taxonomy codes, and required-field errors before the claim reaches the payer.

Corrected Claim vs Adjustment: Which One to Use

When a CO-16 denial arrives, the response is almost always a corrected claim — not an appeal. An appeal argues that the payer's decision was wrong. A corrected claim fixes an error on your end and submits the corrected information for processing. Demographic and data entry denials are almost always your error. Fix it and resubmit.

However, the method of resubmission matters. Submitting a corrected claim incorrectly — as a new claim rather than a replacement — generates a CO-18 duplicate denial. Using the correct billing frequency type code ensures the payer processes the corrected claim as a replacement for the original.

Action	CMS-1500 / 837P Code	When to Use It
Original claim	`Frequency type 1 (or blank — default)`	First submission of any claim. No prior submission exists for this patient/date of service/procedure combination.
Replacement / corrected claim	`Frequency type 7`	A previously submitted claim needs correction. The original claim number must be included in the appropriate field. The payer will void the original and process the corrected version. Use this for CO-16 corrections.

Void / cancel claim	`Frequency type 8`	The claim should be completely voided — no resubmission intended. Used when a claim was submitted in error and should not have been billed at all. Rarely needed for CO-16 situations.

> **INCLUDE THE ORIGINAL CLAIM NUMBER:** When submitting a frequency type 7 corrected claim, the original claim number (the payer's claim reference number from the EOB) must be included in the appropriate field: Box 22 on the CMS-1500 paper form (ICN/DCN field), or the original claim reference number field in the 837P electronic transaction. Without the original claim number, the payer cannot link the corrected claim to the original and will process it as a new submission, generating a CO-18 duplicate denial.

The Human Error Reduction System

Demographic denials are human errors. The most effective way to reduce human errors is not to train harder — it is to design the process so that errors are caught before they cause harm. The following three-layer system applies that principle to medical billing data entry.

Layer 1: Source Verification (Catch Errors at Entry)

Errors enter the system at the moment of data entry. The most effective catch is at the source — before the information is typed into the system.

- Scan insurance cards: a scanned card image attached to the patient record allows anyone who touches the claim to verify the entered data against the source document. Most practice management systems support card image storage. If yours does not, photograph the card and attach the image to the patient file.
- Use structured data entry fields: fields that accept only specific formats (eight digits for date of birth, no letters for member IDs that are numeric-only) prevent the most common transposition errors. Configure your practice

management system to enforce format rules where possible.

- Verify patient identity with a photo ID: for new patients, verify that the name and date of birth in the system match a government-issued photo ID. This catches the common error of a family member presenting for another family member's appointment with the wrong insurance card.

Layer 2: Clearinghouse Scrubbing (Catch Errors Before Transmission)

Clearinghouse claim scrubbing is an automated layer that catches field-level errors before the claim reaches the payer. It does not catch demographic errors (a wrong name passes through scrubbing because the wrong name is still a valid name), but it does catch missing required fields, invalid NPI formats, invalid taxonomy codes, and other structural errors that produce CO-16 denials.

- Enable all available scrubbing rules in your clearinghouse. Most clearinghouses offer basic scrubbing included in their standard service and advanced scrubbing (payer-specific edits) as an add-on. The advanced scrubbing pays for itself in avoided resubmission costs.
- Review the scrubbing report for every batch before transmitting. A batch with scrubbing errors should not be transmitted until the errors are corrected. Transmitting a batch with known errors and hoping some claims go through is a false efficiency.
- Track scrubbing error patterns. The same error appearing repeatedly in scrubbing reports is a workflow problem, not a random mistake. Identify the process step where the error is introduced and fix the process.

Layer 3: Denial Pattern Tracking (Catch Errors After the Fact)

Some errors will get through layers 1 and 2. Layer 3 catches them after the denial arrives and uses the pattern to prevent recurrence.

- Log every CO-16 denial by error type. At minimum: patient name error, DOB error, member ID error, NPI error, referring provider error, POS error, other. A simple tally in a spreadsheet is sufficient.
- Review the log monthly. If one error type appears more than twice in a month: investigate. What caused it? Which staff member entered it? Which patient type or appointment type is most affected? What process change would prevent it?
- Share findings with the front desk. The staff who enter the data are the ones who can prevent the error. They need to know which errors they are making and why. A monthly five-minute review of the CO-16 log with the registration team is more effective than an annual training on everything.

FIX IT: What to do with this denial today

1. Pull the remark code from the EOB. The remark code identifies the specific field that is wrong or missing. Do not attempt to guess or review the entire claim — go directly to the field specified by the remark code.

2. Compare the incorrect field to the source document: the insurance card image, the patient intake form, or the payer's member record in the eligibility portal. Identify the exact error.

3. Correct the specific field in your practice management system. Update the patient record, not just the claim, so the error does not repeat on future claims.

4. Submit a corrected claim (frequency type 7) with the original claim number in the appropriate field. Do not submit as a new claim.

5. Log the error type in your CO-16 tracking log. Note whether this is a recurring error type or a one-time occurrence.

PREVENT IT: What to change so it stops happening

1. Scan insurance cards at every visit for every patient. Store the image in the patient record. This single practice prevents the majority of name and member ID errors because the source document is always available for verification.

2. Run real-time eligibility verification within 48 hours of every appointment and re-verify at check-in. A successful 271 response confirms that the member ID and name in your system match the payer's records.

3. Enable clearinghouse claim scrubbing for required fields and NPI validation. Review the scrubbing report before every batch transmission.

4. Build a CO-16 denial log and review it monthly with the registration team. Patterns emerge within 60-90 days. Fix the process, not just the individual claims.

5. For telehealth claims: create a dedicated claim template with the correct POS code (02 or 10) pre-populated. Telehealth POS errors are among the most common post-2020 CO-16 causes because many practices built their telehealth workflows quickly and the default office POS code was never corrected.

The Front Desk Audit: Finding the Source

When demographic denial rates are elevated and the monthly log review points to a systematic cause, the next step is a front desk audit — a structured review of the registration process for a sample of patients to identify where the error is entering the system.

Audit Question	What You Are Looking For
Is the insurance card being scanned at every visit?	Pull 20 patient records from the prior month and check whether a current card image is on file. If card images are missing or outdated: the scanning step is not being executed consistently.
Is the real-time eligibility check being run before the appointment?	Review the eligibility verification log in your practice management system for the same 20 patients. If verifications are missing or were run at scheduling (not within 48 hours): the verification workflow has a timing problem.
Is the member ID being entered from the card or from verbal patient report?	Ask front desk staff to demonstrate how they enter a new patient's insurance information. If they are typing from verbal report without referencing the physical card: this is the source of member ID errors.

Are staff scanning the entire card or just the front?	The group number is on the back of most insurance cards. If staff are scanning only the front, the group number may be missing or incorrect.
Is the referring provider NPI being stored in the system for frequent referral sources?	Check whether your top 10 referring providers have their NPIs stored in the practice management system's referring provider database. If NPIs are being manually entered on each claim rather than selected from a stored record: transposition errors are likely.

THE 15% RULE: If demographic and data entry denials account for more than 15% of your total denial volume, the practice has a registration process problem, not a billing problem. The fix is upstream. Investing in coder training or billing system upgrades will not reduce CO-16 rates if the data entering the system at registration is consistently wrong. Address the registration workflow first.

> *A name spelled wrong costs as much to fix as a medical necessity denial. It just feels worse because it was completely avoidable.*

CHAPTER 11 · PART 3: SYSTEMS, SPEED & CAREER

The 90-Day Appeal Master Plan

Most practices give up too early — here is the full timeline

The data on denied claims is striking: approximately 60 percent of denied claims are never appealed. Of the 40 percent that are appealed, roughly 65 percent are eventually overturned in the provider's favor. Read those two numbers together and you see the revenue that most practices are leaving on the table — not because their claims are wrong, but because no one followed up.

The reason practices give up is not laziness. It is a lack of a system. When a denial arrives, there is no clear protocol for what to do next, who does it, by when, and what happens if the first attempt fails. So the denial sits in a queue, the appeal window shortens, and eventually the claim is written off.

This chapter provides the system. The 90-Day Appeal Master Plan is a structured timeline from denial receipt through final escalation that covers every step, assigns every action, and gives you the appeal letter templates to execute each stage. It synthesizes the appeal guidance from Chapters 4 through 10 into one repeatable workflow.

Before You Appeal: The 10-Minute Triage

Not every denial is worth appealing. Spending staff time on an appeal that cannot succeed wastes resources that could be applied to winnable claims. Before any appeal is written, run the following 10-minute triage to determine whether the denial is viable.

Triage Question	If Yes — Proceed. If No — Action.
Is the claim amount worth the staff time to appeal?	Rule of thumb: claims under $75 with a low-probability denial type (no documentation, genuine late filing, absolute bundling) are generally not worth a full appeal. Estimate 45-90 minutes of staff time per appeal and compare to the claim value and your estimated overturn probability.
Is the appeal deadline still open?	Every payer sets a deadline for first-level appeals, typically 30 to 180 days from the denial date. Confirm the deadline before drafting. If the deadline has passed: write off and document. If the deadline is within 14 days: escalate to urgent priority.
Is the denial type appealable?	Some denials are not appealable: absolute NCCI bundling edits (modifier indicator 0), genuine timely filing misses with no clock-reset exception, and true plan exclusions for non-covered services with no medical necessity override path. For these: write off. For everything else: continue triage.
Do you have the documentation to support the appeal?	An appeal without supporting documentation has a low overturn rate regardless of how well the letter is written. Confirm you can obtain the relevant medical record pages, payer policy, EOB, clearinghouse records, or prior treatment documentation before committing to the appeal.
Has the root cause been identified?	An appeal submitted without fixing the underlying error is likely to produce the same denial again. Before appealing, identify whether the issue was a coding error (fix and resubmit), a documentation gap (appeal with documentation), or a payer error (appeal with policy argument). The fix and the appeal are separate steps.

The 90-Day Timeline

The 90-day timeline starts on the day the denial is received and received means identified in your denial queue, not the date on the EOB. Every day that passes after denial receipt shortens your appeal window and reduces the probability of recovery. The timeline below assigns actions at specific intervals that keep the appeal on track without letting it stall.

DAY **1**

Denial Identified and Triaged

Read the EOB: identify the reason code, the remark code, and the payer's claim number. Run the 10-minute triage. Classify the denial type (use Chapters 4-10). Log the denial in your appeal tracking system with: denial date, payer, claim number, patient name, denial code, dollar amount, appeal deadline, and assigned staff member.

Outcome target: *Denial classified, viability confirmed, deadline logged, owner assigned.*

DAY **1-3**

Root Cause Determination

Identify the specific error or issue that caused the denial. Pull the relevant documentation: medical record, prior auth confirmation, eligibility verification record, clearinghouse acknowledgment, or original claim. Determine whether the response is a corrected claim resubmission (for coding and data errors) or a formal appeal (for medical necessity, auth, and payer errors). These are different paths with different timelines.

Outcome target: *Decision made: corrected claim path or formal appeal path.*

DAY **1-5**

Corrected Claim Path (if applicable)

For denials caused by correctable errors (wrong modifier, wrong diagnosis, missing NPI, wrong member ID): submit the corrected claim (frequency type 7 with original claim number) within 5 days of denial receipt. Do not wait. Corrected claims are processed faster than appeals and do not consume the appeal window. After resubmission: log the resubmission date and set a 30-day follow-up tickler.

Outcome target: *Corrected claim submitted within 5 days. Tickler set.*

DAY
3-7

First-Level Appeal Drafted and Submitted

For formal appeals: draft the appeal letter using the appropriate template from Section 11.3. Gather all supporting documentation. Submit the complete appeal package to the payer before Day 7. Earlier submission increases the probability of a timely response within the first-level review window. Most payers have 30-45 days to respond to a first-level appeal.

Outcome target: *First-level appeal submitted with full documentation. Response expected by Day 45-52.*

DAY
30

First-Level Appeal Follow-Up

If no response has been received by Day 30: call the payer's provider services line and confirm receipt of the appeal. Get the reference number, the name of the representative, and the expected decision date. Document the call. If the appeal was not received: resubmit with fax confirmation or certified mail and document the resubmission.

Outcome target: *Confirmed receipt. Expected decision date documented.*

DAY
45-
52

First-Level Appeal Response Received

Three outcomes: (1) Approved — post the payment when it arrives. Close the appeal. Document the overturn in your denial tracking log. (2) Denied with explanation — read the denial letter carefully. It should specify which criteria were not met. Use this information to build the second-level appeal. (3) No response — the appeal is deemed denied by non-response in most payer contracts after 45-60 days. Treat as denied and proceed to second level.

Outcome target: *Decision received and processed. Second level initiated if denied.*

DAY
52-
60

Second-Level Appeal or Peer-to-Peer Request

Most payers offer a second level of appeal. For medical necessity denials: request a peer-to-peer review simultaneously with the second-level appeal. Peer-to-peer reviews (physician to payer medical reviewer) have significantly higher overturn rates than written second-level appeals alone. The treating physician must be available for the call within the payer's scheduling window (typically 5-10 business days from request).

Outcome target: *Second-level appeal submitted. Peer-to-peer scheduled (if applicable).*

DAY **75**

Second-Level Response and Escalation Decision

If second-level appeal is approved: post payment, close appeal, document. If denied: assess external review eligibility (see Section 11.4). For high-dollar claims: assess whether legal or contractual remedies are appropriate. For all claims: document the final outcome and root cause in the denial tracking log regardless of result.

Outcome target: *Final internal appeal decision received. External review or write-off decision made.*

DAY **90**

External Review Filing or Final Write-Off

For claims eligible for external review: file the request before Day 90. External review is available for many commercial denials under state insurance law and under the ACA for non-grandfathered health plans. An independent review organization (IRO) reviews the case without deference to the payer's prior decision. IRO overturn rates for medical necessity denials range from 30-60%. For claims not eligible for external review: write off with full documentation of all appeal attempts.

Outcome target: *External review filed or claim written off with complete documentation.*

The Four Appeal Letter Templates

The following four templates cover the appeal scenarios that appear most frequently across the denial types in this book. Each is a complete letter structure — fill in the bracketed fields, attach the specified documentation, and submit. These letters are designed to be direct and brief. A focused one-page appeal with strong documentation outperforms a verbose five-page narrative every time.

TEMPLATE 1: MEDICAL NECESSITY APPEAL (CO-50)

Subject line: *Appeal of Medical Necessity Denial — Claim [#] — Patient [Name] — DOS [Date]*

We are writing to appeal the denial of claim [#] for patient [name], date of service [date], CPT [code], denied as not medically necessary (CO-50). We respectfully disagree with this determination.

The patient presents with [diagnosis/ICD-10], which is identified as a covered indication under [Payer] Medical Policy [policy name/number] or LCD [L-number], Section [X]. The attached clinical documentation dated [date] establishes: [list each coverage criterion from the payer's policy and the specific documentation that satisfies it]. [If step therapy required: Prior conservative treatment was completed as follows: [treatment, date, outcome, attached records].]

This service meets all criteria under the referenced policy. We request reversal and payment of $[amount]. If denied at this level, we request a written explanation identifying the specific criteria not met, and we request a peer-to-peer review with the medical reviewer.

Attach: Relevant medical record pages (highlighted), payer coverage policy or LCD (highlighted), prior treatment records if applicable, supporting clinical guidelines.

TEMPLATE 2: PRIOR AUTHORIZATION APPEAL (CO-24/CO-57)

Subject line: *Appeal of Prior Authorization Denial — Claim [#] — Patient [Name] — DOS [Date]*

We are writing to appeal the denial of claim [#] for patient [name], date of service [date], CPT [code], denied for lack of prior authorization (CO-24). We are requesting reconsideration on the following grounds.

[If retro-auth was obtained: A retroactive authorization was approved on [date], authorization number [#]. The claim should be reprocessed with this authorization number.] [If appealing on medical necessity grounds: The service was medically necessary as documented in the attached clinical records. The patient's condition required timely intervention and the clinical circumstances did not permit advance authorization. Attached documentation supports that all coverage criteria under [Payer] Policy [name] were met at the time of service.]

We request reversal of this denial and payment of $[amount]. Please contact [name] at [phone] with questions or to request additional documentation.

Attach: Retro-auth approval letter (if obtained), relevant medical record pages, payer coverage policy, documentation of clinical urgency if applicable.

TEMPLATE 3: TIMELY FILING APPEAL (CO-29)

Subject line: *Appeal of Timely Filing Denial — Claim [#] — Patient [Name] — DOS [Date]*

We are writing to appeal the denial of claim [#] for patient [name], date of service [date], CPT [code], denied for timely filing (CO-29).

This claim was submitted within the required filing window. Attached is the clearinghouse acknowledgment report confirming that the claim was transmitted on [date], which is within the [X]-day filing requirement applicable to dates of service on [DOS]. [Alternatively: This claim was initially processed as self-pay because insurance information was not available at the time of service. Insurance information was received on [date] and the claim was submitted within [X] days of that date, consistent with your policy for this circumstance.]

We respectfully request that this denial be reversed and the claim reprocessed for payment of $[amount]. Please contact [name] at [phone] with questions.

Attach: Clearinghouse 277CA acknowledgment report, certified mail tracking confirmation (if paper), or portal submission confirmation. Secondary: any payer correspondence or prior EOB relevant to the filing clock exception.

TEMPLATE 4: BUNDLING / MODIFIER APPEAL (CO-97)

Subject line: *Appeal of Bundling Denial — Claim [#] — Patient [Name] — DOS [Date]*

We are writing to appeal the denial of claim [#] for patient [name], date of service [date], CPT [code] denied as included in another service (CO-97).

The service billed under CPT [code] was a separately identifiable [procedure / E/M service] performed [at a different anatomic site / during a separate encounter / for a condition unrelated to the primary procedure], as documented in the attached [operative report / office note]. Modifier [-25 / -59 / -24 / -79] was appended to indicate this distinctness. The NCCI edit table for this code pair (Column 1: [code], Column 2: [code]) has a modifier indicator of 1, indicating the edit is overridable when clinical circumstances support separate billing. The attached documentation confirms those circumstances were present.

We request reversal of this denial and separate payment for CPT [code] in the amount of $[amount]. If denied, we request a written explanation of which element of the clinical documentation was insufficient to support the modifier.

Attach: Relevant medical record pages (operative report or office note with the distinct service highlighted), NCCI edit table printout showing modifier indicator 1 for this code pair.

Second Level and External Review

Most billers stop after the first-level appeal. This is where the significant missed revenue lives. Second-level appeals and external review are underutilized precisely because they require more effort and more persistence — but the overturn rates justify both.

Escalation Level	What It Is	When to Use It

Second-level internal appeal	A second review by a different or more senior clinical reviewer at the payer. Most commercial payers and Medicare have a defined second-level appeal process.	After a first-level denial. Required before external review in most states and under the ACA. Submit within the payer's second-level deadline (often 60 days from the first-level denial).
Peer-to-peer review	A direct phone conversation between the treating physician and the payer's medical reviewer. Not a formal appeal — an informal clinical discussion that frequently resolves medical necessity denials faster than written appeals.	Simultaneously with or immediately after a first-level medical necessity denial. Request at the same time you submit the second-level appeal. Overturn rate with peer-to-peer: 60-70% for appropriate clinical cases.
Expedited appeal	An accelerated first or second-level review for situations where the standard timeline would result in serious harm to the patient. Typically resolved within 72 hours.	When a denial involves an ongoing or imminent service and delay poses a clinical risk. Requires a physician's statement that expedited review is medically necessary.

External / independent review	Review by an independent review organization (IRO) with no financial relationship to the payer. The IRO's decision is binding on the payer in most states.	After exhausting internal appeals. Required to be offered under the ACA for non-grandfathered plans for most denials. State insurance law governs availability for grandfathered and self-funded plans. Most effective for medical necessity denials where documentation is strong.
State insurance department complaint	A formal complaint to the state insurance regulator documenting the payer's denial and the appeal process. Does not guarantee reversal but creates a regulatory record and often prompts a payer response.	When a payer has not responded to appeals within required timeframes, when the appeal process has been obstructed, or when a systemic pattern of improper denials is identified.

EXTERNAL REVIEW ELIGIBILITY: Under the ACA, most non-grandfathered fully-insured health plans must offer external review for any adverse benefit determination. Self-funded ERISA plans are governed by federal external review standards. Grandfathered plans and some state-regulated plans may have different rules. When in doubt about eligibility: call the payer and ask directly whether the denial is eligible for external review. They are required to tell you.

The ROI Decision: When to Write Off vs When to Fight

An appeal that costs more in staff time than the claim is worth is not good revenue cycle management. The following framework helps you make the write-off decision with discipline rather than emotion. The goal is to maximize total recovered revenue per hour of staff time, not to win every individual claim.

Denial Type	Estimated Overturn Rate	Est. Staff Time	Write Off When
Medical necessity (CO-50)	55-70% first level, 60-70% peer-to-peer	60-90 min	Claim under $150, documentation clearly does not support the service, or payer's own policy does not list the diagnosis as a covered indication with no exception path.
Prior authorization (CO-24/CO-57)	30-50% without retro-auth, 70-80% with retro-auth	45-90 min	Retro-auth denied, no emergency exception applies, and claim is under $200.
Bundling (CO-97)	50-60% with correct modifier	30-60 min	NCCI modifier indicator is 0 (absolute bundle), or documentation does not support the distinctness required by the modifier.
Timely filing (CO-29)	70-80% with proof, 15-25% without proof	30-45 min	No proof of timely submission exists and no clock-reset exception applies.

Demographic / data entry (CO-16)	85-95%	15-30 min	Almost never write off CO-16 — the fix rate is too high. Correct and resubmit every time.
Eligibility (CO-31)	40-60% with proof of eligibility at time of service	30-60 min	Verified ineligible at time of service, no proof of eligibility exists, and patient has no ability to pay self-pay amount.

The Appeal Tracking Log

The appeal process is invisible unless it is tracked. Every appeal in progress must have a record that shows its current status, the next action required, and the deadline for that action. Without this, appeals stall and deadlines are missed. The following fields cover everything needed to manage an active appeal inventory.

Field	What to Enter
Patient name + DOS	Identifies the specific claim. Include date of service to distinguish multiple claims for the same patient.
Payer + claim number	The payer's reference number for the original claim. Required for all appeal submissions and follow-up calls.
Denial code + amount	The CO code from the EOB and the dollar amount at stake. Used for ROI triage and priority ranking.
Appeal deadline	The date by which the first-level appeal must be submitted. Calculated from the date of the denial EOB. Flag any appeal within 14 days of deadline as urgent.
Appeal level	Current level: first-level internal, second-level internal, peer-to-peer, external review. Updated as the appeal progresses.

Date submitted	The date each appeal was submitted. Used to calculate expected response dates and follow-up timing.
Response received	The date and outcome of each appeal response: approved, denied with explanation, no response.
Next action + due date	The specific next step and the date by which it must be completed. This is the field that drives the weekly appeal review. If this field is blank or overdue: the appeal has stalled.
Assigned staff member	The person responsible for this appeal. When everyone owns an appeal, no one does.
Final outcome	Paid, written off, or escalated to external review. Documented at case closure. Used for denial trend analysis.

THE WEEKLY APPEAL REVIEW: Review the appeal tracking log every week. Pull every open appeal with a next-action date in the past or within the next 7 days. Execute or escalate. An appeal log that is reviewed monthly is an appeal log full of missed deadlines and unrecoverable revenue. Appeal deadlines do not pause while you are busy.

> *Sixty percent of denied claims are never appealed. Of the ones that are appealed, sixty-five percent are overturned. The math is simple. The discipline required to act on it consistently is the hardest part.*

CHAPTER 12 · PART 3: SYSTEMS, SPEED & CAREER

Denial Rate Benchmarks and KPIs That Matter

How to know if your billing operation is healthy

A billing operation that produces no performance data is impossible to improve. You cannot tell whether this month is better or worse than last month, whether a process change actually worked, or whether a particular payer is generating a disproportionate share of your denial volume. You are managing by anecdote rather than by evidence.

The KPIs in this chapter are the evidence. They are not complex — each one is a ratio or a count that your practice management system can produce with a standard report. What makes them powerful is consistency: tracking the same metrics every month, comparing them over time, and treating a threshold breach as a signal that requires a specific investigation and response.

This chapter covers the four KPIs that matter most, the industry benchmarks to compare against, and the 15-minute weekly dashboard that keeps your billing operation visible.

The Four KPIs That Predict Revenue Cycle Health

These four metrics collectively tell you whether claims are going out clean, coming back paid, being collected efficiently, and being recovered when denied. Any one of them in isolation is incomplete. All four together give you a clear picture of where the revenue cycle is working and where it is not.

KPI 1 Clean Claim Rate	**Formula:** *Claims paid on first submission ÷ Total claims submitted × 100* **Target:** ≥ 95%. A clean claim rate of 95% or higher means fewer than 1 in 20 claims requires any follow-up. This is achievable in a well-run practice and should be the baseline expectation, not an aspirational goal. **Warning threshold:** < 90%. A clean claim rate below 90% means more than 1 in 10 claims is requiring rework. At this level, the billing team is spending a significant portion of its time on claims that should have been paid on first submission. **If threshold breached:** Identify which denial types are driving the rework. Break down denials by reason code for the month. The top two or three codes account for the majority of the gap between actual and target. Address those specific denial types using the relevant chapters of this book.

KPI 2 Denial Rate	**Formula:** *Claims denied ÷ Total claims submitted × 100* **Target:** ≤ 5%. The inverse of the clean claim rate. A denial rate at or below 5% is the industry benchmark for a well-performing billing operation. The national average is approximately 10-15%. **Warning threshold:** > 10%. At this level, the practice is losing significant revenue to denials and spending disproportionate staff time on rework. A sustained denial rate above 10% indicates a systematic process problem, not a series of isolated errors. **If threshold breached:** Segment the denial rate by denial type, by payer, and by provider. A high denial rate from a single payer may indicate a contract issue, a coverage policy change, or a payer-specific coding requirement that has not been addressed. A high denial rate from a single provider may indicate a documentation pattern that needs attention.

KPI 3 Days in Accounts Receivable (AR)

Formula: *Total outstanding AR ÷ Average daily charges*

Target: ≤ 30 days. An AR days figure at or below 30 indicates claims are being paid promptly and the aging is not building up. For practices with a high Medicaid or self-pay mix, a target of 35-40 days may be more realistic.

Warning threshold: > 50 days. At 50+ AR days, a significant portion of outstanding receivables is aging past the point of easy collection. The practice is carrying cash flow risk and facing increasing write-off pressure on older claims.

If threshold breached: Pull the AR aging report segmented by payer type and age bucket (0-30, 31-60, 61-90, 90+ days). Focus first on the 61-90 bucket, which has the highest combination of recovery probability and time urgency. Identify which payers or claim types are driving the aging and address the specific denial or payment delay issue.

KPI 4 Appeal Overturn Rate

Formula: *Appeals overturned in provider's favor ÷ Total appeals filed × 100*

Target: ≥ 55%. An overturn rate above 55% indicates appeals are being filed on viable claims with adequate documentation. Industry benchmarks suggest that well-executed appeals on appropriate claims should achieve overturn rates of 55-70%.

Warning threshold: < 40%. A low overturn rate suggests one of three problems: appeals are being filed on non-viable claims (poor triage), appeal letters are not addressing the specific denial criteria, or documentation is insufficient to support the appeal. All three are fixable.

If threshold breached: Review the last 20 denied appeals. What reason code did the payer give for denying the appeal? Is there a pattern in the denial types that are failing? Are the appeal letters citing the payer's specific policy criteria? Is supporting documentation consistently complete?

Industry Benchmarks: What Good Looks Like

The following benchmarks are drawn from MGMA (Medical Group Management Association) data, HFMA (Healthcare Financial Management Association) standards, and published revenue cycle performance research. Use them as directional targets, not as absolute standards — specialty, payer mix, and patient population all affect achievable benchmarks.

Metric	Best Practice	National Average	Needs Attention
Clean claim rate	≥ 95%	85-88%	< 80%
Denial rate (all denials)	≤ 5%	10-15%	> 20%
First-pass resolution rate	≥ 90%	75-80%	< 65%
Days in AR (overall)	≤ 30 days	35-45 days	> 60 days
Days in AR (commercial)	≤ 25 days	28-35 days	> 45 days
Days in AR (Medicare)	≤ 20 days	18-25 days	> 35 days
Days in AR (Medicaid)	≤ 35 days	40-55 days	> 70 days
AR > 90 days (% of total AR)	< 10%	15-20%	> 25%
Appeal overturn rate	≥ 55%	40-50%	< 30%
Net collection rate	≥ 96%	92-95%	< 88%
Demographic denial rate	< 2% of total claims	3-5%	> 8%
Timely filing denial rate	0% — this should never happen	< 1%	> 1% (any timely filing denial)

NET COLLECTION RATE: Net collection rate measures the percentage of collectible charges that are actually collected. It is calculated as: payments received ÷ (charges billed − contractual adjustments) × 100. A net collection rate below 95% means the practice is not recovering 5 cents of every collectible dollar — a combination of uncollected patient balances, unworked denials, and write-offs that should have been pursued. This is the metric that most directly translates to practice revenue impact.

The 15-Minute Weekly Denial Dashboard

A weekly dashboard does not need to be complex. It needs to be consistent. The following five-report sequence takes approximately 15 minutes to run and review in most practice management systems, and it answers the most important question in revenue cycle management: where is money being delayed or lost right now?

THE 15-MINUTE WEEKLY DENIAL DASHBOARD

Report 1: New Denials This Week

Run: All claims denied in the last 7 days, sorted by reason code. Review: Which denial codes appeared most frequently? Is any single code appearing more than it did last week? A spike in a specific denial code is a process signal, not a random event.

Report 2: AR Aging by Payer

Run: AR aging report segmented by payer, showing balances in 0-30, 31-60, 61-90, and 90+ day buckets. Review: Is any payer's 61-90 or 90+ bucket growing? A growing older-bucket balance from a specific payer signals a payment delay or systematic denial issue with that payer.

Report 3: Open Appeals With Due Dates

Run: All open appeals with next-action dates. Review: Any appeal with an overdue next-action date or a deadline within 14 days is urgent. Assign and act before the week ends.

Report 4: Claims Not Found / No Response

Run: All claims submitted more than 30 days ago with no EOB and no response. Review: These are the claims most at risk for timely filing denials. Check payer portal status for each. If not found: resubmit immediately with proof of original submission.

Report 5: Denial Rate vs Prior Week

Run: Total claims submitted and total denials for this week vs last week. Review: Is the denial rate trending up, down, or flat? A week-over-week increase of more than 2 percentage points warrants investigation. Is a process change responsible? A new payer policy? A new staff member in registration or coding?

Reading the Aging Report

The AR aging report is the most important report in revenue cycle management. It shows every outstanding claim, organized by how long it has been waiting for payment. Reading it correctly — with specific action thresholds for each age bucket — prevents the drift where claims quietly age past the point of recovery while the billing team focuses on new submissions.

Age Bucket	What It Represents	Action Threshold and Response
0-30 days	Claims in normal processing. Most commercial payers adjudicate within 14-30 days.	No action required unless a specific claim shows clearinghouse rejection or no acknowledgment. Monitor, do not intervene.
31-60 days	Claims past standard processing for most payers. Payment should have arrived or denial should have been received.	Check status in payer portal for any claim still showing as pending. If pending: document and monitor. If no record found: initiate status inquiry immediately.

61-90 days	Claims in the follow-up urgency zone. Approaching the appeal deadline for 90-day commercial payer windows.	Every claim in this bucket requires active follow-up this week. Call the payer, confirm claim status, document the call. If denied: initiate appeal immediately. If still pending: escalate to payer supervisor.
91-120 days	Beyond standard processing and approaching or past the appeal window for some payers.	Assess appeal viability for any denied claims in this bucket. Submit appeals immediately for viable claims. For pending claims past 90 days: file a formal inquiry or complaint with the payer. Document everything.
120+ days	Aging that indicates either a systemic payer problem, a process failure, or claims that have been neglected.	Conduct a root cause review of every claim in this bucket. Is this a specific payer that pays slowly? A denial type that was not worked? A timely filing risk? Separate the recoverable from the non-recoverable. Write off what cannot be recovered. Fix the process that allowed the aging to occur.

THE 90+ DAY BENCHMARK: AR older than 90 days should represent less than 10% of your total outstanding AR. When the 90+ bucket exceeds 15-20% of total AR, the practice has a systemic collection or follow-up problem that is eroding revenue month over month. Practices that allow the 90+ bucket to grow without targeted intervention find that a significant portion of those claims become uncollectible — not because the payers refused to pay, but because no one followed up in time.

Payer Performance Scorecards

Not all payers perform equally. Some pay cleanly and on time. Others have high denial rates, slow adjudication, or systematic payment accuracy problems. A payer performance scorecard tracks the behavior of each payer separately, allowing you to identify which relationships are generating disproportionate billing cost and use that information in contract negotiations.

Scorecard Metric	What to Track and Why
Denial rate by payer	Track the percentage of claims denied by each payer separately. A payer with a 20% denial rate while your overall rate is 8% is generating disproportionate billing cost and revenue loss. This data supports contract renegotiation and, in some cases, network participation decisions.
Average days to payment	Track how many days each payer takes from claim submission to payment receipt. Slow-paying payers create cash flow strain. If a payer consistently takes 45+ days while others pay in 14-21 days: this is a contract issue worth raising at renegotiation.
First-pass resolution rate by payer	The percentage of claims paid by each payer on first submission. A low first-pass rate from a specific payer may indicate a payer-specific coding requirement, a coverage policy change, or a systematic issue with how claims for that payer are being built.
Appeal overturn rate by payer	Track what percentage of appeals each payer overturns. A payer with a very low appeal overturn rate may be applying coverage policies incorrectly or using denial as a routine payment delay tactic. Document this for regulatory reporting if the pattern is systematic.

Payment accuracy rate	Compare what the payer paid to what your contract specifies they should have paid. Payment accuracy errors — where the payer paid less than the contracted rate — are common and often go undetected without a contract-rate audit. Even a 1-2% underpayment rate on a high-volume payer represents significant annual revenue leakage.

PAYMENT ACCURACY AUDITS: Most practices verify that payment was received but do not verify that the amount paid matches the contracted rate. Payer payment accuracy errors are estimated to affect 3-7% of all remittances in some analyses. A quarterly audit of 50-100 randomly selected EOBs — comparing allowed amounts to your fee schedule and contract rates — catches systematic underpayments that would otherwise be silently accepted as write-offs.

Putting It All Together: The Monthly Billing Review

The weekly dashboard is operational. The monthly billing review is strategic. Once a month, a 30-45 minute review of the KPI data from the prior month tells you whether the billing operation is improving, stable, or deteriorating – and what to do about it.

MONTHLY BILLING REVIEW AGENDA

1. KPI Review (10 minutes)

Compare this month's four KPIs (clean claim rate, denial rate, AR days, appeal overturn rate) to last month and to the same month last year. Is each metric trending in the right direction? Flag any metric that has moved more than 2 percentage points in the wrong direction for investigation.

2. Top Denial Types (10 minutes)

Review the top five denial codes by volume and by dollar value for the month. Are they the same as last month? Have any new denial types appeared? For each top denial type: identify the root cause, the chapter of this book that addresses it, and the process change that would reduce it.

3. Payer Performance (10 minutes)

Review the payer scorecard for any payer whose denial rate, AR days, or first-pass rate moved negatively this month. Is a specific payer driving outsized denial volume? Has a payer changed a coverage policy without notification? Document and escalate to contract management if the change is systematic.

4. Process Change Review (5 minutes)

Review any process changes implemented in the prior month (new eligibility verification step, modified claim scrubbing rule, updated coding reference). Did the KPIs move in response? If yes: document the improvement. If no: was the change implemented consistently? Was the change sufficient to address the root cause?

5. Next Month Priority (5 minutes)

Identify the single most impactful process change to implement in the coming month based on this month's data. Assign it to a specific person with a specific deadline. One focused change per month, consistently executed, produces more improvement than five simultaneous initiatives that each receive partial attention.

> *A billing operation without KPIs is a billing operation that cannot learn. The metrics do not create performance — they make performance visible. Visible problems get fixed. Invisible ones get worse.*

CHAPTER 13 · PART 3: SYSTEMS, SPEED & CAREER

Modifiers Quick-Reference and Cheat Sheets

Everything you need to keep at your desk

This chapter is a reference, not a lesson. The explanations are in Chapters 2 and 9. What follows is the condensed, desk-ready version — the tables you print, laminate if you are serious about it, and reach for when you are coding a claim, working a denial, or training a new staff member who needs the answer in 30 seconds rather than a textbook explanation.

Four reference tools follow: the 25-modifier at-a-glance table, the payer-specific modifier rules comparison, the 40 most common denial codes with plain-English meanings and first actions, and the EOB remark code lookup for the codes that appear most frequently on denied claims.

13.1 The 25 Modifiers at a Glance

One-line use case for each modifier. When in doubt about whether a modifier applies: read the use case, confirm the clinical circumstance matches, confirm the documentation supports it. If both are true, apply it.

Mod	Name	One-Line Use Case
-21	**Prolonged E/M service**	E/M service required more time than described by the highest-level code in the category (e.g., 99215 exceeded). Use with 99205 or 99215 only.

-22	**Increased procedural service**	Procedure required substantially more work than typically required. Requires documentation of increased complexity. Used sparingly — payers scrutinize heavily.
-24	**Unrelated E/M in postop period**	E/M visit during a surgical global period for a condition unrelated to the original procedure. Required to prevent bundling into global.
-25	**Significant, separate E/M same day as procedure**	A significant, separately identifiable E/M was performed on the same day as a procedure by the same physician. Appended to the E/M code, not the procedure code.
-26	**Professional component**	Only the professional component (physician interpretation) of a service was provided. The technical component was billed separately by the facility.
-32	**Mandated service**	Service was required by a third party (workers' comp, court order, insurer requirement). Waives patient cost-sharing in some payer contracts.
-33	**Preventive service**	Service was provided as a preventive benefit with no patient cost-sharing under the ACA. Applied to specific preventive services to indicate cost-sharing waiver.
-47	**Anesthesia by surgeon**	The surgeon personally administered regional or general anesthesia for their own procedure. Rare use.
-50	**Bilateral procedure**	The same procedure was performed on both sides of the body during the same operative session. Most payers reimburse the bilateral at 150% of the unilateral fee.

-51	**Multiple procedures**	More than one procedure was performed during the same session by the same physician. Appended to the secondary procedure(s). Not used on -51 exempt codes.
-52	**Reduced service**	A service was partially reduced or eliminated at the physician's discretion. Bill for the lesser service actually performed.
-53	**Discontinued procedure**	A surgical or diagnostic procedure was started but discontinued due to extenuating circumstances or risk to the patient's well-being.
-54	**Surgical care only**	The surgeon performed only the surgical portion of a global package. Another provider will perform pre-operative and post-operative care.
-55	**Postoperative management only**	The physician performed only the post-operative care component of a global package. Another provider performed the surgery.
-57	**Decision for surgery**	An E/M service on the day before or day of surgery resulted in the decision to perform the surgery. Prevents bundling of that E/M into the 90-day global package.
-58	**Staged or related procedure**	A procedure was planned at the time of the original service, is more extensive than the original, or is for therapy following a diagnostic service. Used during the global period.
-59	**Distinct procedural service**	Services were distinct due to different session, anatomic site, or separate injury. Overrides NCCI bundling edits when a modifier indicator of 1 applies. Use XE, XS, XP, XU where more specific.

-62	**Two surgeons**	Two surgeons of different specialties operated together as co-surgeons. Each surgeon bills the same procedure code with -62. Payment is split.
-63	**Procedure on infant under 4 kg**	A procedure was performed on a neonate or infant weighing less than 4 kg. Recognizes increased complexity and resource use.
-76	**Repeat procedure, same physician**	The same physician repeated a procedure on the same day. Distinguishes from a duplicate claim.
-77	**Repeat procedure, different physician**	A different physician repeated a procedure previously performed by another physician on the same day.
-78	**Return to OR, related complication**	An unplanned return to the operating room for a complication related to the original procedure, during the postoperative period.
-79	**Unrelated procedure during postop**	A procedure during the postoperative period is unrelated to the original surgery. Prevents bundling into the global package.
-80	**Assistant surgeon**	A physician assisted at surgery. The assisting surgeon bills the same procedure code with -80. Payment is typically 16-20% of the primary surgeon's fee.
-90	**Reference (outside) laboratory**	Laboratory procedures were performed by an outside laboratory. Used when the billing provider is not the performing laboratory.

13.2 Payer-Specific Modifier Rules: Where the Rules Differ

The same modifier does not always work the same way across payers. The following table highlights the most significant payer-specific variations for the modifiers that generate the most denials when applied incorrectly.

Mod	Medicare Rule	Most Commercial Payers	Watch Out For
-25	Accepted. Documentation must show E/M was significant and separately identifiable from the procedure pre-assessment. Audit target.	Accepted by most. Some payers require the E/M to be for a different diagnosis than the procedure. Others accept same-diagnosis if documentation is distinct.	Payers increasingly audit -25 claims. Bundling -25 on every procedure-day visit without distinct documentation generates denials and potential recoupment.
-50	Medicare pays 150% of the single procedure fee for bilateral procedures. Billed on one line with units = 1.	Some commercial payers require two separate lines (one for left, one for right) rather than one line with -50. Confirm the payer's billing format requirement before submission.	Submitting as two lines when the payer expects one line (or vice versa) generates a CO-18 duplicate or CO-97 bundling denial.

-51	Medicare applies MPPR (Multiple Procedure Payment Reduction) automatically. Many Medicare-participating providers do not need to append -51 because the reduction is applied by the system.	Commercial payers vary. Some require -51 on secondary procedures. Others apply their own multiple procedure logic without the modifier. Check each payer's provider manual.	Appending -51 to Medicare claims when MPPR applies automatically can cause payment errors. Know which payer applies the reduction automatically vs manually.
-59	CMS prefers XE, XS, XP, XU over -59 for Medicare claims. -59 remains valid but CMS has promoted the X-modifiers as more specific.	Commercial payers generally accept -59 without requiring X-modifiers. Some have not adopted the X-modifier framework at all.	Using -59 when a more specific X-modifier applies is not a denial risk for most payers, but it increases audit scrutiny for Medicare claims.
-GT	For Medicare, -GT (interactive telecommunications system) has largely been replaced by POS codes 02 and 10 for telehealth billing. -GT may still appear in some Medicare Advantage and state Medicaid policies.	Commercial payers vary widely. Some use -GT, some use -95, some use POS 02/10 without a modifier. Confirm each commercial payer's telehealth billing requirements annually.	Telehealth modifier and POS requirements changed significantly post-2020 and continue to evolve. Always verify current requirements before billing telehealth claims to any payer.

XE/XS/XP/XU	CMS-introduced X-modifiers preferred over -59 for Medicare. XE=separate encounter, XS=separate structure, XP=separate practitioner, XU=unusual non-overlapping service.	Most commercial payers accept X-modifiers but many still prefer -59. A minority of commercial payers reject X-modifiers as unrecognized codes.	Before using X-modifiers with commercial payers: confirm the payer accepts them. If not: use -59 instead to avoid a CO-16 (unrecognized modifier) denial.

13.3 The 40 Most Common Denial Codes

Plain-English meaning and first action for every denial code a biller is likely to see in a typical week. Organized by prefix. Print and keep at the workstation.

Code	Plain-English Meaning	First Action
CO-4	Procedure code inconsistent with modifier or diagnosis	Identify which inconsistency: modifier mismatch or diagnosis-procedure link. Correct and resubmit (coding fix) or appeal (documentation/policy argument).
CO-11	Diagnosis inconsistent with procedure	Check diagnosis-procedure pair. Symptom vs definitive, wrong laterality, or wrong sequencing. Submit corrected claim with appropriate ICD-10.
CO-16	Missing or incorrect information	Read the remark code. It specifies the exact field. Correct the specific field and submit frequency type 7 corrected claim.

CO-18	Duplicate claim	Check payer portal: is the original paid, pending, or denied? Write off duplicate if original is paid. Investigate if original is not found.
CO-22	COB — submitted to wrong payer	Determine correct COB sequence. Resubmit to correct primary payer. Submit to secondary with primary EOB attached.
CO-24	No prior authorization	Check whether retro-auth is available (call payer immediately). If not: appeal on medical necessity. If emergent: appeal on emergency services grounds.
CO-26	Service before coverage effective date	Verify patient's actual effective date. If genuinely before effective date: patient may be responsible. If effective date is in dispute: appeal with enrollment documentation.
CO-27	Service after coverage terminated	Verify termination date. Retroactive termination: appeal with proof of eligibility at time of service. Genuine termination: patient self-pay or write off.
CO-29	Timely filing	Gather proof of original submission (clearinghouse 277CA). Appeal if proof exists. Write off if genuine late filing with no clock-reset exception.
CO-31	Patient not eligible	Verify eligibility for specific date of service. If eligible: appeal with proof. If genuinely ineligible: bill patient or write off per practice policy.

CO-45	Charge exceeds maximum allowable	Routine contractual adjustment. Post as write-off. If allowed amount differs from contract rate: flag for payment accuracy audit.
CO-50	Not medically necessary	Locate the payer's LCD or coverage policy. Write a three-paragraph appeal matching documentation to policy criteria. Attach highlighted medical record.
CO-57	Documentation does not support level billed	Review E/M documentation using 2021 MDM criteria. Appeal with specific MDM elements documented. Request peer-to-peer if available.
CO-58	Treatment was not rendered by appropriate specialty	Verify that the rendering provider's specialty and taxonomy code match the payer's requirements for this service. Correct taxonomy and resubmit.
CO-59	Processed based on multiple procedure rules	A multiple procedure reduction was applied. Verify the reduction percentage matches your contract. If incorrect: appeal with contract rate documentation.
CO-96	Non-covered charge(s)	The service is not a covered benefit under this patient's plan. Verify with payer whether any exception path exists. If not: write off or bill patient depending on ABN/waiver status.

CO-97	Payment included in another service	Identify the bundled code pair in NCCI. Check modifier indicator (0 = no override, 1 = modifier can override). Resubmit with correct modifier if applicable.
CO-109	Claim not covered by this payer	Claim sent to wrong payer. Identify correct payer and resubmit. Common in COB situations where primary/secondary was reversed.
CO-119	Benefit maximum reached	Patient has reached a benefit limit (e.g., number of physical therapy visits). Bill patient for remaining services or obtain new authorization for continuation.
CO-167	Diagnosis is not covered	The specific ICD-10 code is not a covered diagnosis under this patient's plan for this service. Check for a more specific covered diagnosis that the documentation supports.
PR-1	Patient deductible amount	Post to patient balance. Verify the deductible amount against the patient's deductible accumulation on the payer portal. Bill the patient.
PR-2	Patient coinsurance	Post to patient balance. Verify coinsurance percentage matches plan benefits. Bill the patient.
PR-3	Patient copay	Post to patient balance. If copay was collected at time of service: no further action. If not: bill the patient.

PR-96	Non-covered charge: patient responsible	The service is not covered and the patient is responsible. Confirm an ABN or financial waiver was signed. If not: review whether you can legally bill the patient.
PR-204	Not covered by this payer / patient responsibility	Service excluded from coverage. Patient may be responsible depending on ABN/waiver status and your payer contract. Review before billing patient.
OA-18	Duplicate claim — other adjustment	Similar to CO-18 but categorized as an other adjustment. Same investigation process: check payer portal for original claim status.
OA-23	Impact of prior adjudication	Seen on secondary claims. Reflects the primary payer's payment. Verify the primary EOB matches the OA-23 adjustment. Appeal if the calculation appears incorrect.
OA-94	Processed in excess of charges	The payment calculated exceeded the billed amount. Verify the billed amount is correct. Accept the payment — you cannot charge more than the billed amount.
OA-97	Payment included in allowance	Same as CO-97 but categorized as OA. Bundling denial. Same NCCI lookup and modifier correction process.
OA-999	Information required from patient	Payer needs information from the patient (MSP questionnaire, etc.). Notify the patient and provide the payer's contact information and claim reference number.

MA130	Additional information needed (Medicare)	Call the payer and ask specifically what information is missing. The reason code alone is insufficient to identify the field. Document the call.
N30	Patient has other insurance	COB applies. Submit to the other plan as primary and attach the resulting EOB before submitting to this payer as secondary.
N56	Procedure code not on file	The CPT code is not recognized under this provider's contract or credentialing with this payer. Verify credentialing status and contract coverage for this service.
N115	NPI required	An NPI is missing or incorrect. Identify which NPI (billing, rendering, or referring) and correct using the NPPES registry. Resubmit corrected claim.
N130	Consult plan documents	Payer is directing you to the contract or provider manual. Look up the specific policy for the denied service. Appeal with policy reference if the denial appears incorrect.
N382	Invalid patient identifier	The member ID, subscriber ID, or patient name does not match the payer's records. Verify from the physical insurance card and the payer's eligibility portal. Correct and resubmit.

N432	RAC audit finding	A Recovery Audit Contractor has flagged this claim. This requires documentation submission and may involve repayment. Engage a billing compliance specialist for RAC audits.
N517	Resubmit with itemized bill	The payer needs a line-item breakdown of services. Resubmit with an itemized statement rather than a summary claim.
M27	Referral not on file	The referral required for this service is not in the payer's system. Obtain the referral number from the referring provider and resubmit with the referral authorization number.
M76	Missing/incomplete/invalid diagnosis	The diagnosis code field is missing, invalid, or incomplete. Identify the specific code issue (deleted, non-specific, missing) and submit a corrected claim.

13.4 Global Period Quick Reference

The global period is the time window following a surgical procedure during which the post-operative care is included in the procedure's payment. Billing separately within the global period without the correct modifier produces CO-97 or CO-4 denials. This table covers which modifier to use for which situation.

Global Period	Applies To	Included in Global	Modifier to Separate

0-day global	Minor procedures (e.g., laceration repair, shave biopsy, destruction of lesion)	Day of surgery and any E/M on the day of service related to the procedure.	Modifier -25 on the E/M if a significant, separate E/M was performed on the same day for a different or additional condition.
10-day global	Minor procedures with brief follow-up (e.g., incision and drainage, simple fracture care)	Day of surgery plus 10 days of routine post-operative care.	Modifier -24 (unrelated E/M), -78 (return to OR for related complication), -79 (unrelated procedure during postop period).
90-day global	Major surgical procedures (e.g., joint replacement, appendectomy, laparoscopic cholecystectomy)	One day before surgery, day of surgery, and 90 days of routine post-operative care.	Modifier -24 (unrelated E/M), -57 (decision for surgery E/M), -58 (staged/related procedure), -78 (return to OR related complication), -79 (unrelated procedure).

0-day global—same-day rule	Any 0-day global procedure billed with a same-day E/M	The pre-procedure assessment is bundled. A separate E/M requires documentation of a significant, separately identifiable service.	Modifier -25 on the E/M. Documentation must clearly separate the E/M content from the procedure pre-assessment.

13.5 Place of Service Codes at a Glance

An incorrect place of service (POS) code is one of the most common causes of CO-16 denials and payment rate errors. The POS code affects not only claim validity but also the Medicare payment rate — facility-rate vs non-facility-rate reimbursement differs significantly for many services.

POS	Setting	When to Use	Medicare Rate
11	**Office**	Services rendered in the physician's private office, clinic, or group practice office.	Non-facility rate (higher)
12	**Home**	Services rendered in the patient's private residence (not an assisted living or nursing facility).	Non-facility rate
02	**Telehealth — patient not at home**	Synchronous telehealth where the patient is at a location other than their home (e.g., a clinic or originating site).	Facility or non-facility depending on the originating site

10	**Telehealth — patient at home**	Synchronous telehealth where the patient is located in their home. Post-COVID expansion broadened this POS significantly.	Non-facility rate
19	**Off-campus outpatient hospital**	Hospital outpatient services rendered at an off-campus provider-based department (not the main hospital campus).	Facility rate (lower for physician)
22	**On-campus outpatient hospital**	Hospital outpatient services rendered at the main hospital campus or a qualifying provider-based department.	Facility rate (lower for physician)
23	**Emergency room**	Services rendered in a hospital emergency room.	Facility rate
24	**Ambulatory surgical center**	Surgical procedures performed in a Medicare-certified ambulatory surgical center.	Facility rate (lower for physician)
21	**Inpatient hospital**	Services rendered to a patient admitted as an inpatient to a hospital.	Facility rate
31	**Skilled nursing facility**	Services rendered to patients in a Medicare-certified skilled nursing facility.	Facility rate

32	**Nursing facility**	Services rendered in a non-Medicare SNF nursing facility.	Facility rate
65	**End-stage renal disease treatment facility**	Dialysis services rendered at a dialysis facility.	Facility rate

> **FACILITY VS NON-FACILITY RATE:** When a physician performs a service in a facility setting (hospital, ASC, outpatient department), the facility bills separately for the overhead, staff, and equipment. The physician's payment is reduced (facility rate) because those costs are covered by the facility's claim. When a physician performs the same service in their own office, they bear all costs — so the payment is higher (non-facility rate). Using the wrong POS code can result in the physician being paid at the facility rate when the non-facility rate applies, or vice versa. The POS code on the claim must match the actual location of service.

13.6 Billing Frequency Type Codes

Frequency type codes tell the payer whether a claim is an original submission, a corrected replacement, or a void. Using the wrong frequency code is the most common cause of CO-18 duplicate denials when resubmitting corrected claims.

Code	Name	When to Use	Original Claim # Required?
1	**Original claim**	First submission of any claim. No prior submission exists.	No
6	**Corrected claim (institutional / UB-04)**	Corrected version of a previously submitted UB-04 inpatient or outpatient hospital claim.	Yes — include in FL 64

7	**Replacement of prior claim (CMS-1500 / 837P)**	Corrected version of a previously submitted physician claim. Voids the original and processes the corrected version. Use for all CO-16 corrections on physician claims.	Yes — include original ICN/DCN in Box 22
8	**Void / cancel of prior claim**	Complete cancellation of a previously submitted claim. No resubmission intended. No payment should have been made, or an overpayment must be returned.	Yes — required to link to original

THE MOST IMPORTANT RULE IN THIS CHAPTER: Modifier -25 belongs on the E/M code. Not on the procedure code. Modifier -59 (or the X-modifiers) belongs on the component service being separately billed. Not on the comprehensive service. Modifier -50 goes on one line with units of 1, not on two lines. These three errors account for the majority of modifier-related CO-4 and CO-97 denials. If you remember nothing else from this chapter, remember the placement rule for -25, -59, and -50.

CHAPTER 14 · PART 3: SYSTEMS, SPEED & CAREER

Remote Work and Career Path in Medical Billing

How to get hired, work remotely, and grow

Medical billing is one of the few healthcare careers that has been fully remote-compatible since before remote work became mainstream. The work is computer-based, the output is measurable, the systems are cloud-accessible, and the patient interaction is administrative rather than clinical. Practices have been hiring remote billers for decades, and the post-2020 expansion of remote work infrastructure has made it easier than ever to build a career in this field from anywhere.

This chapter is honest about what that career looks like — the realistic entry points, the salary ranges at each stage, the certifications worth obtaining and the ones worth skipping, where legitimate remote jobs are found and where scams concentrate, and the three specialties that pay significantly above the general biller rate. It ends with a career path map that shows where the first job leads and how long each stage typically takes.

The Realistic Salary Picture

Salary data in medical billing varies significantly by geography, experience, credential level, specialty, and employer type. The following ranges are drawn from BLS Occupational Employment data, MGMA compensation surveys, and AAPC salary surveys. They represent what the market actually pays — not what job postings advertise and not what certification programs promise.

Role / Level	Median Annual	Range (25th–75th percentile)	What Gets You to the Top
Entry-level biller (0-2 years, no credential)	$36,000–40,000	$32,000–45,000	Employer, geography, willingness to learn quickly. Remote roles often pay slightly below on-site for entry-level.
Medical biller (2-5 years, certified or experienced)	$44,000–50,000	$40,000–58,000	Certification (CPC, CPB, CBCS), specialty experience, demonstrated denial reduction results.
Senior biller / denial specialist (5+ years, specialty-focused)	$52,000–65,000	$48,000–75,000	Specialty expertise (see Section 14.5), appeal win rate, ability to train others, multi-payer proficiency.

Billing manager (team lead, 7+ years)	$65,000–85,000	$58,000–$100,000+	Management experience, KPI ownership, revenue improvement track record, multi-provider or multi-specialty oversight.
Revenue cycle director (large practice or health system)	$90,000–$130,000	$80,000–$160,000+	Breadth of system knowledge, P&L accountability, vendor management, contract negotiation experience.
Independent billing contractor / small billing company	Varies: $25–45/hour or % of collections	$40,000–$120,000+ depending on client volume	Client acquisition, reputation, specialty focus, ability to manage multiple accounts simultaneously.

> **REMOTE VS ON-SITE SALARY:** Remote roles for entry-level billers often start $2,000-$5,000 below on-site equivalents because employers factor in eliminated commute costs and the lower cost of living in many remote workers' locations. At the senior and manager level, remote roles frequently match or exceed on-site equivalents because the talent pool is national and top performers command market rates regardless of geography. The salary gap narrows significantly with experience and specialization.

Certifications Ranked by Value

The certification landscape in medical billing is crowded with options that range from genuinely valuable to essentially worthless. The following ranking is based on employer recognition in job postings, salary premium data from AAPC and AHIMA surveys, and the practical utility of the credential content for actual billing work.

Rank	Credential	Issuing Body	Who Should Get It and Why
1st	**CPC (Certified Professional Coder)**	AAPC	The most recognized coding credential in outpatient physician billing. Opens more doors than any other billing or coding certification. If you plan to work in physician practice billing for any length of time, this is the credential to pursue. Requires passing a 150-question exam and 2 years of experience (or 1 year with a training program).

2nd	**CPB (Certified Professional Biller)**	AAPC	Billing-specific credential that validates knowledge of the full revenue cycle, denial management, and payer-specific rules. More directly focused on billing than the CPC (which is coding-heavy). Ideal for billers who are not pursuing a coding role but want a recognized credential. Can be obtained without 2 years of prior experience.

3rd	**CBCS (Certified Billing and Coding Specialist)**	NHA (National Healthcareer Association)	Entry-level credential that is widely accepted by employers as evidence of baseline competency. Faster to obtain than CPC or CPB. Appropriate as a first credential for someone new to the field who wants to begin working while building toward a more advanced certification.
4th	**CCS (Certified Coding Specialist)**	AHIMA	More relevant for hospital/facility coding than physician billing. High value in the inpatient coding market. If you intend to work in hospital revenue cycle or health information management rather than physician practice billing, CCS is the preferred credential over CPC.

5th	**CMRS (Certified Medical Reimbursement Specialist)**	AMBA	Less widely recognized than the above credentials. Has value in demonstrating general billing competency but carries less weight in job postings than CPC, CPB, or CBCS. Consider only if you have already obtained one of the higher-ranked credentials.

Not recommended	**Online certificates from non-accredited programs**	Various	Numerous programs sell 'medical billing certificates' for $200-$2,000 that are not recognized by employers. These are not the same as certifications from AAPC, AHIMA, or NHA. Before paying for any program: verify whether the issuing organization is AAPC, AHIMA, or NHA. If not: research employer recognition before enrolling.

> **WHICH CERTIFICATION FIRST:** If you are choosing between CPC and CPB for a first credential: CPB is faster to obtain and more directly aligned with billing work. CPC requires more study time and covers coding in depth that may exceed what a billing-focused role requires. However, CPC opens more doors in the long run because many employers treat it as the standard baseline for any revenue cycle role. If time and study resources allow: pursue CPB first to start working, then CPC within 12-18 months to maximize opportunity.

Where to Find Legitimate Remote Jobs

Remote medical billing jobs exist in volume. The challenge is separating the legitimate postings from the scams that concentrate in this field, and knowing which employers and platforms consistently produce real opportunities.

Legitimate Sources

- Indeed.com and LinkedIn: the highest volume of legitimate remote billing job postings. Search terms: 'medical biller remote,' 'denial management specialist remote,' 'revenue cycle remote,' 'AR specialist remote.' Filter by posted date (within last 7 days) to avoid stale postings.
- AAPC Career Center (aapc.com/medical-coding-jobs): postings targeted specifically at credentialed billing and coding professionals. Lower volume than Indeed but higher relevance. Employers posting here expect to hire certified candidates.
- AHIMA Career Center (ahima.org/careers): more focused on health information management and coding, but includes revenue cycle and billing management postings at mid to senior levels.
- Physician practice management companies and revenue cycle management (RCM) companies: large RCM companies including Optum360, Conifer Health, R1 RCM, Greenway Health, and Athenahealth frequently hire remote billers at scale. Applying directly through their careers pages yields opportunities that do not appear on job boards.
- Hospital system careers pages: most large health systems (HCA, Tenet, CommonSpirit, AdventHealth, etc.) hire remote billing and AR staff at scale. Their careers pages list current openings and allow direct application.
- Physician practice referrals: experienced billers often find their best remote opportunities through professional referrals. If you know someone working in billing at a practice that hires remotely, a referral is the most effective job search tool available.

Scam Warning Signs

HOW TO IDENTIFY A MEDICAL BILLING SCAM: Work-from-home medical billing scams are among the most common in the healthcare job market. Red flags: (1) The 'employer' requires you to purchase software, equipment, or training materials before you can start working. Legitimate employers provide or reimburse these. (2) The job pays a percentage of billings with no base salary and the 'clients' are provided to you by the company. This is almost always a pyramid structure. (3) The posting guarantees income of $50,000+ with no experience required and no credentials. (4) The hiring process involves no interview, no skills assessment, and an immediate offer. (5) Payment is requested from you before employment begins, for any reason. Real employers pay you.

The Remote Work Setup: What You Actually Need

Most employers who hire remote medical billers provide or specify the software and systems you will use. What they expect you to provide is a home office environment that meets their security and productivity standards. The following covers what most remote billing employers require and what you need to invest in before applying for remote roles.

Requirement	Details and Employer Expectations
Computer	Most employers require a PC (Windows) rather than Mac, because most practice management systems and clearinghouses are Windows-optimized. A laptop with at least 8GB RAM, a current processor, and 256GB storage is the practical minimum. Some employers provide a company laptop — confirm before purchasing.

Internet connection	High-speed broadband (minimum 25 Mbps download, 10 Mbps upload). Many employers require wired Ethernet connection rather than Wi-Fi for security and reliability. A wireless router with an Ethernet port and a cable to run to your workstation is a $30-50 investment that prevents most connectivity denial issues during work hours.
Second monitor	Remote billing work involves simultaneously viewing a payer portal or EOB on one screen and your practice management system or claim on the other. A second monitor is not optional for sustained productivity. It is also frequently the single biggest efficiency investment a remote biller can make.
Private workspace	HIPAA compliance requires that patient health information (PHI) not be visible to unauthorized individuals. Your workspace must be in a room with a door that can be closed. Open-plan apartments shared with family members or roommates who can see your screen do not meet HIPAA standards for remote billing work.
VPN / secure access	Most employers provide their own VPN or remote access solution. Do not install personal VPN software on an employer-provided device without explicit authorization. For your own equipment: confirm the employer's VPN requirements before purchasing.
Quiet environment	Not a formal requirement but a practical one: billing work involves calls with payer representatives, follow-up calls, and peer-to-peer review phone calls. A consistently noisy home environment affects professionalism on calls and concentration during complex claim work.

Three Specialties That Command Premium Rates

General outpatient billing — primary care, family medicine, internal medicine — is where most billers start. It is also where the most competition for positions exists and where the salary ceiling is lowest. Three specialty areas consistently pay above the general biller market, and the reasons are the same across all three: the coding is more complex, the denial management requires specialized knowledge, and fewer qualified billers are available.

Specialty	Why It Pays More	What You Need to Learn First
Oncology / infusion billing	Chemotherapy drug billing (J-codes) is one of the most complex areas in all of medical billing. Drug coverage policies change frequently, prior authorization requirements are extensive, waste and overfill billing rules are payer-specific, and the per-claim dollar values are high. A billing error on a chemotherapy infusion can represent thousands of dollars. Employers pay for precision.	J-code structure and drug billing basics, Medicare Part B vs Part D drug coverage distinctions, infusion code selection (96413-96417 primary and additional hours), the CMS Oncology Care Model reporting requirements, and payer-specific overfill and waste billing policies.

Behavioral health / mental health billing	Mental health parity laws, complex prior authorization requirements, note length and content requirements for session-level billing, telehealth-specific billing rules, and coverage limits that vary dramatically by plan make behavioral health billing a specialized skill that general billers typically cannot perform without specific training.	CPT codes 90791-90899 (psychiatric diagnostic evaluation, psychotherapy, medication management), parity compliance basics, place of service rules for telehealth mental health (which expanded significantly post-2020), and payer-specific documentation requirements for session-by-session medical necessity.
Orthopedic surgery / surgical billing	High procedure volume, complex global period management, extensive use of surgical modifiers (-62, -80, bilateral procedures), implant and supply billing, and high-dollar denied claims make orthopedic billing a specialty where precision directly translates to revenue. The per-claim values are high, the modifier rules are complex, and denial rates are elevated when coding is imprecise.	The global surgical package in depth, surgical modifier decision trees (-22, -50, -51, -58, -62, -78, -79, -80), implant and supply pass-through billing, hospital vs ASC billing differences for the same procedure, and the post-2023 E/M changes for surgical encounters.

THE FASTEST PATH TO SPECIALTY BILLING: You do not need to start in a specialty to work in one. Most specialty billers started in general outpatient billing and moved into a specialty when an opportunity arose. The transition typically requires 6-12 months of focused self-study in the specialty's coding and billing rules, ideally while working in a general billing role. AAPC offers specialty-specific credentials (COSC for orthopedic surgery, COC for oncology coding) that demonstrate specialty competency to employers and command salary premiums.

The Career Path Map

Medical billing careers follow a relatively predictable progression when the biller is intentional about skill development and credential acquisition. The following map shows the typical stages, the realistic time at each stage, and what moves you to the next level. It is not a guarantee of timeline — it is a realistic picture of what deliberate career development looks like in this field.

STAGE 1: ENTRY LEVEL (0-18 months)

Role: Medical billing clerk, billing assistant, AR entry-level. Starting in a physician practice, medical billing company, or hospital billing department. Learning: the practice management system, the payer portal, basic claim submission, and payment posting.

Priority actions: obtain CBCS or CPB within the first 12 months. Build familiarity with your practice's top 5 payers and their specific denial patterns. Keep a personal denial log of everything you see and how it was resolved.

STAGE 2: WORKING BILLER (18 months – 4 years)

Role: Medical biller, billing specialist, AR specialist. Independently managing a claim queue, working denials, submitting appeals, and monitoring aging. You know your payers, your denial types, and your practice's billing patterns.

Priority actions: pursue CPC if you have not already. Begin tracking your personal KPIs: your clean claim rate, your denial rate, your appeal overturn rate. These numbers are your professional portfolio. Consider specialization: identify the specialty that your current employer or the local job market values most.

STAGE 3: SENIOR SPECIALIST (4-7 years)

Role: Senior biller, denial management specialist, AR manager, specialty biller. You have a measurable track record: denial rates reduced, appeal overturn rates documented, system improvements implemented. You are training junior billers and being consulted on complex denials.

Priority actions: formalize your results. Build a one-page summary of your KPI improvements: 'Reduced denial rate from 14% to 7% over 18 months. Appeal overturn rate of 68% on medical necessity denials.' This is the document that justifies a significant salary increase or a management promotion. If you are interested in management: begin taking on training and mentorship responsibilities now.

STAGE 4: MANAGEMENT OR INDEPENDENCE (7+ years)

Two paths diverge here. The management path leads to billing manager, revenue cycle director, or VP of revenue cycle — roles that involve team leadership, vendor management, and P&L accountability. The independent path leads to independent contractor or billing company owner — working for multiple physician clients, owning your schedule, and earning based on volume and results rather than salary.

The management path requires demonstrated leadership experience and the ability to own metrics across a team. The independent path requires client acquisition skills, business administration basics (contracts, invoicing, taxes for self-employed), and the discipline to manage multiple client relationships simultaneously. Both are viable. The choice depends on whether you want to build an organization or build a business.

Starting Independent: The Basics

Independent medical billing is one of the few genuine work-from-home businesses with a real market, real clients, and real income potential. It also has real risks and real startup requirements. The following covers what you need to know before leaving an employer-based role.

- Experience requirement: most independent contractors who sustain viable billing businesses have 5+ years of experience and at least one specialty credential. Practices hire independent billers because they want expertise, not entry-level learning. Starting as an independent biller with less than 3 years of experience and no specialty focus is difficult.

- Pricing models: the two most common are a flat fee per claim (typically $3-$8 per claim depending on complexity) or a percentage of collections (typically 4-8%). Percentage-based pricing aligns your incentives with the practice's revenue — you are paid more when you collect more. Flat-fee pricing is more predictable for budgeting. Know which model the practice prefers and which aligns with your workflow.
- Contract: always work under a written contract. At minimum: scope of services, payment terms, access to the practice management system and payer portals, HIPAA Business Associate Agreement (required), and termination terms. Do not start work without a signed BAA. Handling PHI without a BAA is a HIPAA violation regardless of how small the practice.
- HIPAA Business Associate Agreement: as an independent contractor who accesses patient health information, you are a Business Associate under HIPAA. The practice must provide a signed BAA before you begin. If they are unfamiliar with this requirement, explain it — it protects both of you.
- Software access: confirm which practice management system the practice uses and verify you can access it remotely. Some older systems do not have cloud access and require remote desktop software. Factor setup time into your onboarding estimate.
- Client acquisition: the most effective method for small billing operations is direct outreach to small physician practices that are currently billing in-house with staff who manage other administrative functions. These practices often underperform on claims because billing is a secondary priority. A conversation about denial rates and first-pass performance often opens the door.

The Long-Term Skill Stack

The billers who command the highest rates and the most career flexibility over a 10-to-20-year horizon are not the ones who simply processed more claims. They are the ones who built a skill stack that extends beyond claim submission into the areas that practices and health systems are willing to pay premium rates for.

Skill Area	Why It Commands Premium Pay
Denial analysis and process improvement	The ability to identify the root cause of systematic denial patterns, implement process changes, and document measurable KPI improvement is the highest-value skill in revenue cycle management. It is rare, it is directly tied to revenue, and it is what separates a billing manager from a billing clerk.
Contract rate verification and underpayment recovery	Auditing EOBs against contracted rates and identifying systematic underpayments is a billable service that most practices either do not perform or outsource to specialized firms. A biller who can perform this audit generates direct, measurable revenue recovery.
Payer credentialing and enrollment	Credentialing new providers, managing re-credentialing cycles, and enrolling providers with new payers is an administrative bottleneck in every growing practice. Billers who add credentialing to their skill set can offer a more complete revenue cycle service.
Compliance and audit preparation	Knowledge of RAC audits, OIG work plans, and documentation requirements for high-risk services (E/M upcoding, modifier overuse, medical necessity) allows billers to help practices reduce audit risk. This is a consulting skill that commands consulting rates.

Revenue cycle software proficiency	Deep expertise in specific practice management systems (AdvancedMD, Kareo, athenahealth, eClinicalWorks, Greenway) is valued by employers and clients who use those systems. Being the person who knows the system best — including reporting, configuration, and workflow optimization — makes you difficult to replace.

> *The medical billing career that pays well at every stage is not built on volume. It is built on outcomes — on the documented ability to reduce denials, recover appeals, and improve the revenue numbers that practices care about. Build that record from day one.*

www.ingramcontent.com/pod-product-compliance
Lightning Source LLC
LaVergne TN
LVHW010720061126
851857LV00014B/1282